SKINNY DIPPING IN THE FOUNTAIN OF YOUTH

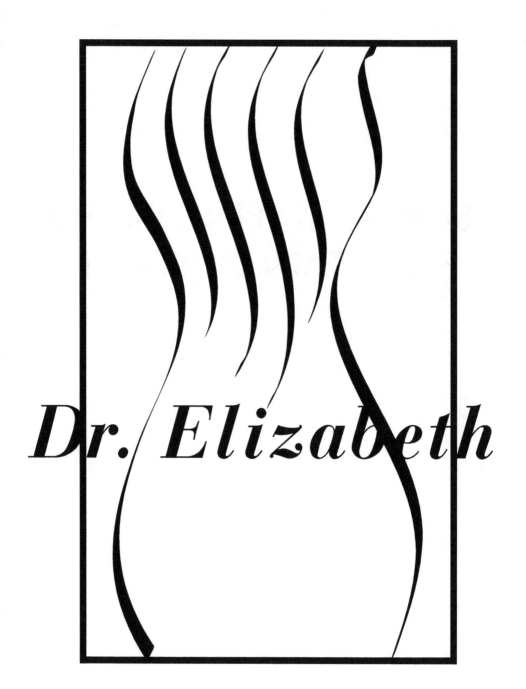

SKINNY DIPPING

in the

FOUNTAIN

of

YOUTH

How to be UNDENIABLY Radiant, Beautiful,
Youthful and Sexy at Every Age.

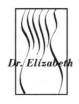

Dr. Elizabeth

This book is written as a source of information only. The contents contained in this book should not be considered a substitute for the advice of a qualified physician or qualified medical professional and cannot replace the diagnostic expertise, medical advice and/or treatment of a trusted physician. Always consult a physician or qualified medical professional before beginning any new diet, exercise, therapeutic regimen and/or health or lifestyle program, particularly if you suffer from any medical condition or have any symptom that may require treatment. The author and the publisher expressly disclaim responsibility for any adverse effects arising from the use or application of the information contained herein. The publisher and author are not responsible for any adverse reactions to the recipes contained in this book. References are provided for informational purposes only and do not constitute endorsement of any websites or other sources. Some names in this book have been changed to protect the privacy of the individuals involved.

This book may be purchased for educational, business, or sales promotional use. For more information please write to Speaker@DrElizabeth.com or visit www.DrElizabeth.com

FIRST EDITION

Designed by Harrison G. McKoy

Library of Congress Cataloging-in-Publication Data has been applied for.

ISBN 978-0-692-34583-2

*This book is dedicated to each one of you beautiful souls
who has the courage to reach for and live from
your greatest self. May your journey be paved with grace, ease
and fun, and your life be filled with love, laughter and joy.*

And
*To my beloved mother, Lucille, who has been my greatest
supporter. You have taught me through your own example the
true meaning of love.*

Contents

Introduction

Welcome, I am so delighted and honored that you are here with me and thrilled to share this exciting adventure with you. It is my heart's deepest desire that this book contribute something beautiful to your already divinely kissed life.

I offer this book from my heart to yours, may it be of service to you in some way. May it give you a piece of the puzzle that you've been searching for, an answer to a question that has been dancing in your mind, your heart or your spirit. May it feed a stirring that has been flickering in your soul.

I fought writing this book for several years, struggling with the daunting and isolating process of putting my thoughts onto paper. Even when a clairvoyant whom I'd never met before, tapped me on my shoulder and pronounced, "You're going to write a book that is going to help a lot of people someday." I graciously responded with a somewhat bewildered smile and a look like, "You've got to be kidding me, buddy. Me? A writer? No way."

However, what began happening is that, as I met people and shared what is in my heart and how I have been living my life, they began asking for my book. It took awhile for me to surrender to the process. I'm much more comfortable on stage in front of thousands of people than I am alone with my computer. I receive and translate the downloads that Spirit flows through me far more easily and rapidly when face to face with other human beings than I do when I am in the company of myself.

So it's perfect that this book was an act of courage for me, because, as I share these seven keys with you, it may be an act of courage for you to embrace and incorporate them into your life.

I call these seven secrets in my book keys because they open, not a door, but a powerful gateway that has the capacity to transport you directly to the fountain of youth.

I call it skinny dipping because being radiant, beautiful, youthful and sexy at every age is fun, exciting and incredibly freeing. To fully reap the benefits of frolicking in the fountain of youth, you must first get naked from the inside out. That means throwing aside your inhibitions and stripping off what no longer serves you so that your true beauty, light and essence can shine through. This is the real secret to becoming undeniably and eternally gorgeous.

Do you ever wonder why some people never seem to age? It's as if they have an all access pass to the fountain of youth. Have you ever secretly wished you could slow down or even reverse the aging process in your own life?

There is a kaleidoscope of factors involved in remaining forever youthful. Most of them have much more to do with what is going on inside your body rather than outside. You might be surprised to learn it's easier than you think to be forever, stunningly radiant and ageless.

The idea of skinny dipping in the fountain of youth is absolutely fascinating to me. With all the extraordinary technology offered today coupled with brilliant new discoveries in quantum physics, science and a greater awareness of ancient spiritual wisdom, it makes perfect sense that we could improve and extend the health and life force of our physical bodies. And why not, we live in an ever-expanding Universe of infinite possibilities.

My entire life I have been intrigued by the idea of human potentiality and the infinite abundance of the Universe. The subjects of health, fitness, nutrition and spirituality captivate me. Growing up, I was enthralled and inspired by the question, "How much can we expand the love in our hearts, the heights our spirits can soar, the strength our bodies can achieve, the depths our souls can reach and the genius and creativity our minds can express?"

I've always had the sense that we all have the capacity to be so much more than we are currently expressing. Over the years, I've gone on an adventure to test my theory. I decided to use myself as an experimental laboratory to test what foods give us the most energy, what movements help keep us strong and flexible, what practices allow our hearts to give and receive the most love, what thoughts open us up to our genius capacity and what ways of being allow us to flourish and soar.

What I observed along the way is that we truly do have the capacity to literally grow younger, stronger, deeper, richer, wiser, more flexible, more beautiful, more expansive, more radiant… better in every way.

Through my explorations I believe that I've discovered the equivalent of the modern day fountain of youth. This fountain is real, and it is rich in magic and miracles.

"WHAT I WANT MOST IN MY LIFE IS TO BE THE GREATEST MANIFESTATION OF MY BEING."
–*Oprah Winfrey, Talk Show Host, Entrepreneur and Humanitarian*

The full expression of a human being's capacity is their radiance. Webster's Dictionary defines radiance as "Emitting rays of light, shining, vividly bright, expressive of and bright with joy, hope, love, confidence, happiness."

At the essence of your core, you are Light. Light is the highest frequency in the Universe. When you are truly living the greatest manifestation of your being; body, mind, heart, soul and spirit, you are absolutely and undeniably radiant and youthful.

Radiance transcends beauty. It goes far beyond the constructs of age, color or physical appearance. It is the full expression of light and love.

What I realize as I continue to circle the sun each year, another way of saying aging, is that the by-products of living fully in your radiance are greater:

- Energy
- Enthusiasm
- Eternal Beauty
- Freedom
- Fulfillment
- Youthfulness
- Sex Appeal
- And much more…

This Book will help you:

- Get in better shape and stay in shape
- Discover your passion for yourself and life again
- Look years younger
- Get your glow on
- Have more confidence
- Be gorgeous from the inside out
- Create a greater, deeper and more delicious sex life and a fuller expression of your sexuality and sensuality

It will help you uncover and rediscover your:

- Innocence
- Creativity
- Artistry
- Imagination
- Passion
- Unconditional Love
- Deepest desires for your life

You'll automatically begin to manifest a stronger, healthier, sexier more youthful body, have more energy and vitality, feel better, have more peace, discover and foster richer, more beautiful and fulfilling relationships, earn more money and create or cultivate a wonderful loving intimate relationship.

Think of this book as a buffet. You can feast on the entire menu or just sample individual chapters as they call to you. Either way works perfectly to transport you directly to the sweet, healing and rejuvenating waters of the fountain of youth.

Now that we've discovered the secret gateway, grab your key and let's step through the portal into chapter 1, CHOICE.

Choice

CHAPTER 1

Choice

The first step in becoming more radiant, beautiful, youthful and sexy at every age is to have the courage to be open to the possibility of saying yes.

It has been said by numerous spiritual teachers that we are spiritual beings having a human experience. As human beings, we have free will. Unlike birds that fly south for the winter out of instinct, we must continuously and consciously choose our path, our thoughts and our actions.

Change begins with choice and choice begins with willingness. If you are open to the possibility of saying yes where you have previously said no, real change can occur. Here's the beauty about willingness, you don't even have to say yes. Your willingness is enough. Once you open up, Spirit steps in and miracles occur.

Three Words that Changed My Life Forever

My entire life I dreamed of being a dancer. The visions in my meditations were so real that I physically felt the experience of dance in every cell of my body. That cellular memory was reminding me of the gift of dance that's been encoded deep within my soul for many lifetimes.

Since I didn't have the opportunity to study dance as a child, by the time I reached my late 30's I thought that "the dance ship" had sailed and I "missed the boat." I even used to joke that next lifetime I was going to come back as a dancer to fulfill my dream.

One day, a dear friend of mine took me to see a powerful clairvoyant. She uttered three words that changed the course of my life forever.

The woman took one look at me and proclaimed, "You're a dancer." I quickly assured her I was not.

But then something so magical happened that it set my life on a brand new trajectory. There was something in the tone of her voice, the way she looked at me and the power and grace of Spirit flowing through her that woke me up from my logic-induced slumber.

In a flash, I caught the vision she was seeing of my destiny. There was something in the way she looked at me that caused the most miniscule opening to occur in my heart. Inside of that opening, a miracle occurred.

You see, if I say no, there's nothing spirit can do. The door is sealed shut. Remember, we have free will. Our angels and Spirit guides cannot override that. But even in the slightest opening, Spirit can rush in and work its magic.

This is exactly what happened for me. Very serendipitously, soon after my experience with the clairvoyant, a friend invited me to go dancing with her at "The Coconut Club." This was the late 1990's and "The Coconut Club" was the chicest place to go swing dancing. I walked in the club and the dance floor was packed with incredible dancers. Men were tossing their dance partners into the air with the greatest of ease and executing intricate aerials and fancy footwork with delicious perfection.

Then, as if by sheer magic, one of the male dancers appeared next to me. From somewhere deep inside me, before I had the chance to think it through, I blurted out, "Will you do a lift with me?"

Our dreams have very little to do with thinking and the logical process of the mind. Before I knew it, I was flying through the air squealing with delight!

After he set me down and I regained my composure, he mentioned that there was a gentleman at the club who owned a swing dance company. He proceeded to tell me that they perform all over the country and suggested I introduce myself to him.

Before he even finished his sentence, I made a beeline over to the gentleman, introduced myself and declared my passionate desire to join his dance company.

He replied, "Well kid, I have more than enough girls on the team already. What I really need are guy dancers. If you know any male dancers, send 'em over." Then he spun around on his heels and scurried away.

My heart plummeted to the floor as my dream was momentarily dashed. Then I took a breath. Understand that the Universe can speak to us in a millisecond when we just center ourselves and breathe. In that moment Spirit whispered to me, "Just ask if you can go to the rehearsal anyway." So that is exactly what I did. He responded, "Suit yourself kid, but you're wasting your time."

That Saturday I showed up for rehearsal, dance shoes in hand. The team was preparing for a dance performance that evening for an environmental event Ted Danson was hosting at the Beverly Wilshire Hotel. Shortly after rehearsal began, one of the girls got sick. Since there were no other girls at the rehearsal, the owner turned to me in a panic and implored, "Can you learn two swing dance routines and perform with the company this evening?" I replied with tremendous glee, "You bet I can."

One of the other girls in the dance company brought a beautiful costume for me to wear. That night I got to break in my brand new pair of official dancing shoes in my very first professional dance performance. I was forty years of age at the time.

Once I went from being an absolute no, to just being open to what Spirit wanted to create for me and through me, I found myself on stages performing with dance partners half my age and fulfilling one of my lifelong dreams, being a professional dancer.

If you think about it, it makes absolutely no sense for a woman to begin a dance career with no prior dance training at the age of 40.

But the expression of our life's purpose rarely has anything to do with logic. Never, ever allow your logical mind to muffle out the songs in your heart. They are there to encourage you to follow your dreams and remind you to share your unique gifts with the world.

To this day, dancing is one of the greatest joys in my life. I can't imagine living without it. In addition to the tremendous joy and fun I experience, many people have been inspired to follow their heart's deepest desires after hearing my story and seeing me perform on stage.

Following your heart's purpose and joy has powerful and uplifting ramifications on the lives of others in ways you can't possibly imagine. To think that I have had the blessed opportunity to inspire others to pursue their purpose is a privilege that is beyond comparison.

Exercise #1 Choose to Follow Your Heart's Desires

What is one dream in your heart that you could begin to awaken and cultivate right now? If you can't think of one, look back at what you did as a child. What were the activities that captivated your attention and passion for hours on end? Make a list of these activities even if they seem completely illogical and nonsensical.

For example:

- Paint pictures
- Newspaper route
- Play with make up
- Play let's pretend

- Cut your hair (or someone else's hair)
- Create a lemonade stand
- Play with Lego blocks
- Build model airplanes
- Read books
- Sit quietly and observe while the other children play

Now make a list of activities you dream of doing now.

For example:

- Take a painting class
- Learn to sing
- Start of business
- Go back to school
- Take photographs
- Write a book

Make a play date, either alone or with friends and choose to do one of those activities again. See how it makes you feel. Watch how alive you become. And if you have children, do this exercise with them. It's amazing how much fun you'll have together.

You may be wondering how these childhood activities could possibly help you discover and follow your heart's desires today. What in the world could a paper route possibly have to do with your life's purpose? Well, if you were business savvy enough to manage a paper route, lemonade stand, snow shoveling, lawn mowing or baby-sitting service as a child, you are a born entrepreneur.

These childhood activities and secret dreams are clues that can lead you to your divine purpose. Like golden threads, when you follow them, they guide you to your life's purpose encoded in your heart. When you engage in these adventures, they reveal what you most deeply desire to share with the world.

Begin to incorporate these activities into your life on a regular basis. When you make room in your life and in your schedule for your dreams, they have the ability to present themselves to you in unique and miraculous opportunities. When they do, get out of your logical mind with its limitations and just say YES.

Zero Point... Infinite Possibility

Quantum physics tells us that at every moment we are at zero point-infinite possibility.

That sounds great, but what does that actually mean? Simply put, it means that at every moment, we have at our disposal a limitless number of choices. What we choose impacts the way we experience our life.

Here is a story that illustrates this concept perfectly.

Flipping the Switch

"BOREDOM IS THE EFFORT IT TAKES TO SQUELCH YOUR CREATIVITY."
–*Dr. Michael Beckwith, Spiritual Teacher and Author of "Spiritual Liberation"*

Rose is a single, 42 year old account executive who commuted an hour to and from work every day. She tolerated her job because it paid the bills but somewhere in her heart she longed for more. Lately Rose had noticed that she'd gained a few pounds and it was a little more difficult than usual to lose the excess weight. She also noticed that she found herself bored with her life and her passion for fun and adventure had waned. She couldn't remember the last time she got dressed up, went out with friends and had fun or was asked out on a real date.

After a long day, she'd come home, pop a frozen dinner in the microwave, sit down and mindlessly allow the television to watch her. Then she'd get up the next morning feeling fuzzy and dull, pour herself a cup of coffee, in an attempt to wake up and do it all over again.

Then one day Rose was flipping through a magazine and something caught her eye. She felt a sensation in her body that she hadn't felt in a very long time, enthusiasm. It was an advertisement for a scuba diving class at the local community college. At first Rose hesitated to follow up on the ad, but something in her heart egged her on. Before she knew it, her fingers anxiously dialed the phone number and a voice appeared on the other end of the line. "Hello?" Rose took a deep breath. For a split second she contemplated hanging up the phone. Her mind berated her, "What in the world is a 42 year old woman who barely swims and hasn't exercised in years doing signing up for a scuba class?" But, in that breath she heard something whisper to her, "Just say hello." Rose replied, "I wanted to know about the beginner scuba diving lessons you're offering at the college." The women said, "You're just in time, today is the last day to sign up and we have one spot left in the class. It's your lucky day." Rose's fears waned a bit as she took another deep breath, "Okay, I'll sign up."

That is how Spirit operates. Rose had the courage to make the call and life created a space in the class just for her. Little did she know at that moment, this class would also be an opening for a remarkable new life.

The moment Rose plunged into the pool her first night of class she felt at home. She secretly longed to learn how to scuba dive since she was a little girl, but never took the time to engage in something so frivolous for herself. It was a thrilling evening. She even met a wonderful woman named Laurie and they became fast friends.

Since the course was quite physically demanding, Rose decided to start working out at the gym. She invited Laurie to join her at the gym the nights that they didn't have scuba diving class. Soon Rose began noticing that her body was getting stronger, leaner, more agile and more flexible. Nutritious food choices replaced frozen dinners and a healthy lifestyle quickly ensued.

Rose and Laurie were so passionate about their newly acquired skill that they signed up for a scuba diving trip to Costa Rica.

This story is a great example of what I call "Flipping the Switch." Just by making the choice to follow her passion and take a scuba diving class, Rose's entire life shifted for the better.

It doesn't matter which expanded choice you make, as long as you make one. All healthy roads lead to the same place. Rose could have just as easily decided to sign up for the gym first, or take a healthy living foods preparation class. The point is that once you alter one behavior, the others follow suit. It would have been impossible for Rose to continue sitting on the couch each night mindlessly watching TV, eating unhealthy foods and stay in her scuba diving class. Her body needed to build up the strength necessary to swim with heavy tanks on her back. The dead food dinners (more about living foods in chapter 3- FOOD) would not have nourished Rose's physical body enough to allow her to engage in the strenuous activity of scuba class.

Remember the point of the story, at every moment we are at zero point, infinite possibility. The choice to come home, consume a non-nutritious meal and check out for the evening took Rose on a downward spiral of weight gain, boredom, isolation and depression. The simple choice to sign up for a scuba diving class put Rose on an expansive and upward spiral of excitement, weight loss, friendship, better health, stronger, leaner, sexier body and a desire to engage with the world.

But that's not the end of the story. Rose and Laurie had such an incredible time on their scuba diving adventure that they promptly signed up for a scuba diving teacher's certification program class upon their return. Each evening after class or the gym, they would grab a healthy bite to eat at a local restaurant and talk about their passion for scuba diving. Because of their desire to travel to tropical destinations to dive and teach others how to do the same, they caught a beautiful vision to create a company that takes people on scuba diving adventures all around the world. This little side project of theirs became so popular and expansive they soon quit their dull jobs and led exciting scuba adventures full time. They even met the loves of their lives on one of their journeys. That's what happens when we Choose to follow our heart's desires.

Choose Your Thoughts Wisely

"CHANGE YOUR PERCEPTION OF AGING… SAY TO YOURSELF, EVERYDAY, IN EVERY-WAY I'M INCREASING MY PHYSICAL AND MENTAL CAPACITY, BECAUSE YOU CAN."
–Deepak Chopra, Spiritual Teacher, Physician and Best Selling Author

On a daily basis I hear people say, "I'm getting old." Men and women of all ages lament about this.

It's Time for a New Conversation

Saying you're getting old has incredibly damaging effects on your body as well as your spirit. If you tell yourself that your body is getting old, where is there any possibility of growing young?

There is absolutely no room for expansion when your mind and consciousness are engaged in constriction. If you are truly interested in becoming more youthful, vital, sexy and radiant, begin shifting your pre-programmed thoughts and subsequent words on aging.

Scientific evidence now proves that when the cells of your body hear these messages, they begin to breakdown. When you shift your thoughts from disempowering, low vibration messages to empowering, high vibration messages, the cells of your body respond accordingly and you begin to turn back the hands of time.

Exercise #2 Choose to Speak to Yourself Differently

I invite you to make the choice right now to start speaking to yourself in ways that are empowering.

Awareness is the first key. Start by listening to yourself. I know that might sound silly, but if you will begin to listen to the way you speak to yourself, the thoughts you think, the words you say, you will cultivate a new way of communicating with yourself and others that is much more empowering.

Before you go to sleep at night, tell yourself, "Tomorrow I will speak kindly to myself and about myself." This plants the suggestion, like a potent seed, deep into your subconscious. Then write yourself a little reminder note and put it by your alarm or cell phone or on your nightstand (if you don't use an alarm). Here's an example of what the note might say:

"Good Morning Beautiful. You are healthy, radiant and youthful. Today you are going to speak kindly to yourself and about yourself all day long."

When you wake up in the morning, before you get out of bed, you will see this love note reminder and consciously make a different choice in the ways you speak to and about yourself.

Do this practice for twenty-one days and watch those old belittling comments fade and new more empowering comments emerge. The reason I invite you to do this for twenty one days is because this is the amount of time scientists say it takes to engrain a new habit into our daily routine.

It's All Over After 35

I have the great privilege of dancing on stage with women and men who are young enough to be my children. These individuals are in their 20's and 30's and it astonishes me to hear them say, "I'm over the hill." I tell all of them, "NO, not so. At 55 years young, I'm just getting started and I'm here to remind you that the sky's the limit for all of us!"

Many of these young women and men are incredibly talented singers, actors and dancers in the entertainment industry. Their greatest fear is that they won't be able to realize their dreams before becoming what society considers "too old." It's as if there is an omnipresent "age police" patrolling the streets ready to "out" anyone who is past their "teenage prime."

Just like in the movie, "The Wizard of Oz," it's time to pull back the curtain and expose this illusion. The notion of "getting old" is an insidious lie that has been programmed into our subconscious and into the fabric of our society.

It's time to smash this pervasive mass consciousness that says, "You're over the hill. Your body is breaking down. You look old. You can't do the same things that you used to be able to do when you were younger…etc., etc., etc."

One of the reasons I continue to dance on stage is that I want to be a reminder to others that you can do anything your heart desires at any age, no matter the circumstances.

Here's a brilliant demonstration that you're never too old to realize your dreams. In 2009, at almost 50 years young, Susan Boyle took the stage as a contestant on "Britain's Got Talent." As she introduced herself and shared her dream of becoming as grand a star as Elaine Paige, the entire audience scoffed at her. However, so strong was Susan's self-assurance that as she prepared to sing her first note, she donned a cheeky smirk as if to say, "You might be laughing at me now, but just you wait and see. Give me two notes and I will instantly change your tune." Stunning everyone, including Simon Cowell with her performance of "I Dreamed the Dream," she inspired each and every skeptic to their feet in a massive standing ovation.

Today, fans all over the world are still cheering her to the tune of 25 million records sold worldwide. This from a woman who, prior to appearing in "Britain's Got Talent" was single and unemployed, in her late 40's, living in a tiny Scottish village with her cats.

Don't let the world rob you of your dreams. Just as Susan dug deep and chose to stand in her self-confidence, I invite you to stand up and share what it is that you have to give to others.

Begin today to shift your thoughts to those that expand you. Tell yourself, "I'm getting better everyday. I'm committed to being stronger, younger, deeper, more flexible, more beautiful and more radiant." You'll be amazed that when the body hears these messages, it will, quite literally, follow suit.

In addition, as you reprogram your thought patterns you will be inspired to make choices that support this new way of thinking and being; choices such as picking foods that nourish you, engaging in healthy exercise, being grateful, meditating and associating with people who contribute to your life and who you contribute to in their life.

Falling Prey to "The Infallible Years"

"YOUTH IS WASTED ON THE YOUNG."
–*Oscar Wilde, Writer and Poet*

There is a misconception surrounding youth that I call, "The Infallible Years." Learning to navigate this time period with a few simple tools allows you to mine the gifts that youth provides and enjoy youthful radiance throughout your life.

"The Infallible Years" is that time period when you can eat whatever you want, pull all nighters, drink and party to your heart's content and still wake up, as Carrie Bradshaw from "Sex and the City" once said, "Stunning and impossibly fresh looking."

Because of the illusion that "The Infallible Years" will continue indefinitely, many people fall prey to the misconception that they can prolong the abuse forever, and their bodies will just continue to naturally bounce back. Unfortunately, however, this is not the case.

For most, "The Infallible Years" last throughout their teens and twenties. For a lucky few it can even carry over into their late thirties. However, by their late forties, nearly everyone has outgrown "The Infallible Years."

For men, the six-pack turns into the fat pack. For women, the changes can be even more brutal. Their once strong lean thighs get soft and chubby and their tight tummies turn to jelly. There are other permutations as well. Bright youthful radiant skin turns sallow, wrinkled and lack-luster.

In addition, people's energy levels begin to wane, as do their coordination skill levels. Where they once could easily play several basketball games on a Saturday afternoon, now, they're winded half way through the first game. Their jumps aren't nearly as strong, their shots are weak and off balance and they're just off their game.

One day they find themselves running up a flight of stairs at work and they are shocked to discover that they can't catch their breath. A simple physical task that used to be effortless becomes strenuous.

If they continue down this path of destruction, eating junk, drinking excessively, partying and staying up all night, before they know it, they don't even recognize their reflection in the mirror. This person wonders what in the world happened and asks, "Where did that beautiful, vibrant person go? Seems like just yesterday I was youthful, full of energy and enthusiasm."

This is when, where and why most people begin to say the three most deadly words anyone wanting to tap into the fountain of youth could ever utter, "I'm getting old."

Once an individual mutters those fateful words, it's a rapid and slippery slope to old age. Most people don't realize the profound damage that is done to the cells of their body when they declare, "I'm getting old."

Year after year I witness friends transform from healthy, strong, vital bodies to overweight, under energized, weakened bodies.

It breaks my heart to see these unnecessary shifts happen to people simply because they didn't make healthier choices. The dangerous truth is that the conscious or unconscious decision to neglect the wellbeing of their body affects every other aspect of their life including career, life purpose, health, relationships, sex, marriage… everything.

Most people take better care of their homes, cars and clothing than they do their bodies. This is the only body you get this lifetime. The wisest and most significant decision you can ever make is to take care of it. Remember, a tiny bit of prevention is worth a pound of cure when it comes to the health and well being of your body temple.

The good news is that these physical challenges are completely avoidable and reversible. There are ways to navigate "The Infallible Years" with awareness so that instead of shriveling into the sunset, by actively incorporating the following steps, you can continue to enjoy the rich juiciness and radiant sex appeal bestowed upon the young.

Steps to maintaing your juicy youthfulness after "The Infallible Years":

- Embrace the awareness that "The Infallible Years" won't last forever.
- Remember that it's the simple daily choices that create health and wellbeing.
- No matter what your age, start loving your body and feeding it foods that are nourishing (see chapter 3 FOOD).
- Get enough rest every day. Most people need between 7-8 hours of sleep each night.
- If you enjoy yourself a little too much the night before, take some time to rejuvenate the next day.
- Drink lots of purified water to help flush out toxins.
- Begin to incorporate physical, emotional and mental detox techniques (see chapter 2 HEAL).

When you practice these simple tips, you can enjoy a lifetime of youthful radiance. Here's a powerful story that demonstrates this point perfectly.

"I'M MAKING LONG TERM PLANS FOR MY LIFE."
–Bernando LaPallo, Longevity Expert, Author of "Age Less, Live More"

In 2012, I had the great privilege of speaking at the Raw Spirit Festival in Scottsdale, Arizona. On stage, one of my fellow presenters enthused that

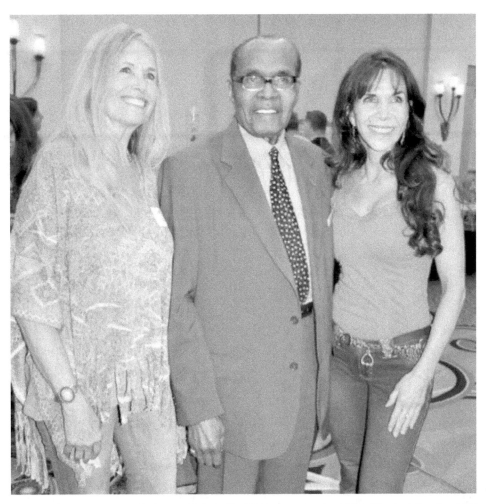

Mimi Kirk (76 years young), Bernando LaPallo (113 years young) and Dr Elizabeth Lambaer (55 years young), all raw (living food) vegans.

he's making long-term plans for his life. Nothing earth shattering about that these days, except for the fact that Bernando LaPallo is 113 years young this year! (Birth date: August 17th, 1901)

Strong, sharp, bright, funny and more alive than most people 1/4th his age, this man had the energy and vitality of a teenager.

Bernando shared with his audience that he is enthusiastically making plans to open a raw food restaurant in Mesa, Arizona soon. This is not a man who in any way, shape or form thinks he's getting old. Quite the contrary, everything about him is youthful, vibrant and alive.

He attributes his longevity to healthy living foods, exercise and a proper mindset. The incorporation of these practices causes an expansive upward cycle. The more you think of yourself as young, vibrant, youthful and healthy, the better choices you make.

I invite you to follow in Bernando's footsteps and start making long term plans to grow younger every time you circle the sun. It's certainly working for him.

Exercise #3 Long Term Plans

Make a list of 25 things you'd like to do in your lifetime. Think of it as your bucket list. Be ambitious and outrageous. It's just as easy for the Universe to deliver a bottle of water as it is an all expenses paid trip around the world, so think big.

When making your list, don't ask yourself, "How could I possibly do that?" Just write down the things that you've always dreamed of doing. Let the Universe surprise you with its magical manifestations. You're just in charge of allowing your heart to tell you what it most deeply desires and then writing it down on your list.

For example, maybe you've always dreamed of going to France and learning to speak French. Don't let your logical mind berate you with questions such as, "How in the world are you ever going to manage to pull that off?" or "Don't be so unrealistic, you can't just up and move to France." Just write it down and stay in the energy of infinite possibilities. Let the Universe handle the details.

For all you know, you or your beloved could suddenly be transferred to Paris for work. Or you could manifest a brand new job in the south of France. Just be open to the miracles that the Spirit can provide.

Maybe you've always dreamed of taking a cruise around the world. Or perhaps you want to go back to school or start a business. I invite you to fill this chart with all of the things that make your heart sing.

- _____
- _____
- _____
- _____
- _____
- _____
- _____
- _____
- _____
- _____
- _____
- _____
- _____
- _____
- _____
- _____
- _____
- _____
- _____
- _____
- _____
- _____
- _____
- _____
- _____

The Beauty Game

Society places a great deal of focus on the external shell. Now, in my opinion, there's nothing wrong with wanting to improve and maintain your physical appearance. It's a well-known fact that when people look younger and better, they feel younger and better.

However, placing your attention solely on making the exterior more attractive isn't the way to true beauty. You may have smooth, taut skin, but you'll never be luminous.

The irony is that when you choose to switch your primary focus from external beauty to internal radiance, you actually become exponentially more beautiful, physically and in every other way.

An Array of Exquisite Beauty

You can't open up a fashion magazine without being bombarded with images of what the media considers beautiful. In an era where fashion models are 5'10", 110 lbs and 12 years of age, what kind of message does that send to women?

No offense if you're very tall and very thin, but that is not the only sample of what's beautiful. Personally, I am incredibly grateful to Beyoncé and Jennifer Lopez for owning and flaunting their beautiful sexy curves. As a woman who was teased for being " too curvy" growing up, I celebrate the diversity in woman's shapes, sizes and colors. It's important to remember that beauty comes in an array of exquisite expressions.

Owning Your Undeniable Beauty

Several years ago I taught a "Sexy Dance Class" at the Learning Annex. There were approximately 60 women in the class. We were dancing in a very large dance studio lined with mirrors. I recall standing in front of the classroom, teaching the women how to sway their hips side to side and being blown away by the unique allure of each and every woman in that class. It was a veritable buffet of beauty.

There were women of all shapes, sizes, colors and ages. As the women began to discover and express their feminine sensuality, they became stunningly gorgeous and undeniably sexy.

Youthfulness and radiance occur when you begin to own your unique beauty and inner luminosity and have the freedom to express it fully.

Bless Every Compliment No Matter What

Not too long ago I had the great pleasure of meeting a very striking, young African woman, Nana from Ghana, in the gym. She's a model, actress and artist whose beautiful spirit captured me from the moment we met. She is stunning physically with a body that could stop traffic, but it is her inner light and spirit that makes her truly gorgeous.

During our first encounter she relayed a story about an annoying experience she had with a man who was trying to pick her up at the gas station. Aghast, she rolled her eyes with disgust as she shared her exasperating experience.

I asked my new friend if I could share something with her from my heart, something that could help her be even more beautiful than she already was. She cordially consented.

I said, "Nana, the day you stop getting compliments is the day you should be annoyed. At 55 years young, I bless and appreciate every single compliment I receive. My philosophy is that no matter how awkward the comment, I choose to see the person who gave me the compliment as showing appreciation for my radiance. And for this, I am tremendously grateful." Nana smiled, gave a nod of approval and said, "That's a great idea, thank you for the gift."

I have seen many beautiful women act "put upon" when a man gives them a compliment. I often wonder what happened to those same women once the compliments began to wane. Did they ever wish they had been more gracious and grateful for the attention that their beauty gravitated to them in their youth?

There are some people in the world that would give anything for just one compliment, once in their life. Bless and appreciate every single compliment you receive. Even if the person who is giving it appears to have ulterior motives, even if you're not interested in them. You don't have to stay and talk with them, you don't have to give them your number or go out on a date with them. You can simply say, "Thank you for the blessing of my compliment." This way you always remain gracious and grateful.

There is an added benefit to this practice. When you see the comment being given to you as a great blessing you raise not only the energy of the words being given to you, but also the energy of the person who is sharing those words.

Let's say the man or woman giving you the compliment has a hidden agenda of some sort and you're not interested in them. By blessing the words and the person speaking them, you literally transform the energy from a low level to a high level frequency.

I have left many a man scratching his head wondering what I had just done when I responded, as I kept on walking, "Thank you so much for the blessing of my compliment," to his, "Hey baby you're so hot, wanna go in the back room with me right now?"

The energy of grace and gratitude vibrates at a very high frequency. A woman or man who comes from this place will always be stunningly beautiful, no matter what their age. If you want to be showered with genuine compliments until the day you leave this earth, make the decision to bless every accolade that comes your way.

The choice is yours. Choose wisely. The power to create the life of your dreams is in your hands. Now that you have opted in, the next step is to HEAL.

Heal

CHAPTER 2

SKINNY DIPPING IN THE FOUNTAIN OF YOUTH

Heal

The second key to becoming undeniably radiant, beautiful, youthful and sexy is to heal.

What I have discovered is that even before putting healthy nourishment into the body, it is imperative to first release the toxins that you have accumulated over the years.

Cleansing is a continual process of releasing what no longer serves you. This can be done physically, emotionally, mentally, spiritually and in relationships.

The greatest gifts detoxing gives you are expanded awareness and consciousness, which, in turn, allows you to make the choices that naturally and effortlessly bring increased beauty, radiance and youthfulness.

Think of your body as an instrument. The universal life force cannot flow through you when it is clogged with toxic waste, mental garbage, emotional baggage and rigid dogma.

Make Your Saxophone Sing

One beautiful Sunday at Agape International Spiritual Center, my beloved spiritual community founded by my dear friend, Dr. Michael Beckwith, the choir was singing and the house band was rocking. As I was enjoying this delicious artistic feast, I observed my friend, LaDonna's husband, world-class saxophone player, Cal Bennett performing on stage. In that moment, I had a thought. What if Cal's saxophone was filled with junk? As brilliant a musician as he is, if his saxophone is clogged, try as he may, he cannot make that instrument sing.

The same thing holds true for your physical instrument. If your body is encumbered with poisonous toxins, negative thoughts, dead food waste and chemicals, the Universe cannot sing its exquisite song through you.

So how can you get and keep your saxophone clean?

Physical Healing

"WHAT WE TAKE OUT OF OUR BODIES IS EVEN MORE IMPORTANT THAN WHAT WE PUT INTO OUR BODIES."
–Markus Rothkranz, Raw Food Expert and Author of "Heal Yourself 101"

Let's begin with physical cleansing. If you've been consuming a standard American diet (S.A.D) affectionately referred to as the SAD diet, most likely your intestines are congested and you are not absorbing a lot of nutrients. Even if you start consuming healthy living foods, until your intestines are unclogged, your nutritional absorption rate remains low.

For those of you who are already consuming a raw vegan diet, which in my opinion is the most effective way to garner nutrients, it is still important to do a physical detoxification (detox/cleanse) on a regular basis.

Your environment is loaded with pollution, radiation, electromagnetic frequencies from your cell phone and technical devices and many other toxins. A cleanse will help clear out these pollutants and allow your body to operate at maximum efficacy.

So, What is a Body Detox and How Can You Start this Process?

Quite simply, it is a detoxification process designed to clear toxins out of your pipes (intestines) so you can absorb the greatest amount of nutrition.

If you are dealing with a serious illness, or if you just want to take the "Evelyn Wood speed detoxing" fast track, the following techniques are fabulous ways to efficiently and effectively clean your body of toxic waste:

- Enemas
- Colonics
- Fasts- affectionately called "Juice Feasts"

If you want to take a more gentle and scenic route to a cleaner, healthier physical body, these methods are great:

- Internal body cleansers
- Living foods juices and smoothies (more about this in chapter 3 FOOD)

"YOU RELEASE ABOUT 60% OF YOUR ACCUMULATED WASTE IN THE FIRST SEVEN DAYS OF A CLEANSE!"
–*Kris Carr, Wellness Activist and Author of "Crazy Sexy Diet"*

Now, I am very well aware that some of these methods may sound a bit radical. I invite you to do what you feel is best for your own body, health and healing.

When you're in the midst of your detox, and you're asking yourself, "Why in the world am I doing this?" just remember, the results you'll get from physical cleansing are far better than anything the best plastic surgeon could ever deliver...with much less pain and a much more palatable price tag.

What are the Benefits of Doing a Cleanse/Detox?

You'll feel lighter, cleaner, clearer, stronger and brighter. You'll have exponentially more energy and greater access to your intuitive capacities.

Your skin will have a remarkable glow to it and you will look years younger. Don't be surprised if people start asking you, "Why do you look so amazing? What did you do? Are you in love?"

Detoxing in combination with a living foods lifestyle, which I'll describe in the next chapter, is a powerful combo to keep you looking like you skinny dip in the fountain of youth on a daily basis.

NOTE: Consult your physician or health care professional before participating in, or proceeding with any detoxification or cleansing program.

I offer a reference section for this book on my website www.DrElizabeth. com. There you will discover a list of wonderful books, detox programs, products, services and other valuable resources that will assist you in your detoxing journey.

Mental Detox

Every dis-ease in the body has a mental and emotional component. Clear away the mental and emotional toxicity and you'll help heal the body.

Our thoughts can be as toxic to our souls as bad food is to our bodies. As you clean out your physical body of toxins, take time to cleanse your mental body of negative thoughts.

Exercise #4 Methods for Clearing Out Mental Toxins

- Download a recording app on your phone, or get a tape recorder, and record everything you say for one day.
- At the end of the day, listen to the recording. You may be shocked at some of the negative words that come out of your mouth.
- Listening to the recording will give you a better idea of what you are thinking throughout the day.
- Once you are aware of what you are thinking and saying, you can begin to catch yourself and make changes in your thought patterns

and your language.

- Keep a journal for a week and record your positive thoughts and words each day.
- Reward yourself every time you choose a healthy word or thought over a negative one.
- Ideas for rewards can include going to the movies, buying yourself something nice, taking a walk, getting a massage or whatever feels like a treat to you.

The key to this exercise is to become conscious of your negative thoughts, and begin to shift them to more empowering thoughts.

Psychoneuroimmunology

Psychoneuroimmunology is the scientific study of the effect of the mind on health and resistance to disease. In other words, what we think and feel has a tremendous impact on the health, vitality and continued youthfulness of the physical body.

There are numerous books written on this subject. I mention it here to scientifically substantiate my premise that as you choose to practice these detoxification methods, shift your thoughts and begin to see yourself as radiant and youthful, your physical body will quite literally follow suit.

Emotional Detox

An equally important part of the cleansing and clearing process is emotional detoxification. Negative emotions, such as anger, shame, guilt, hatred, jealousy and revenge vibrate at a low frequency and cause immense damage to the cells of your body.

There is No Selection Button on Emotions

There are numerous factors that can cause someone to suppress their emotions. It can stem from parental disapproval of the expression of negative emotions, such as anger, fear of being hurt or any number of other circumstances. Regardless of the reason, when you suppress one emotion, that action shuts down the expression of all of the other emotions.

For example, if you sit on your anger, and don't freely and fully express it, that will cause you to unconsciously suppress your joy, love and all the other positive emotions as well.

Almost everyone has shut down one or more of their emotions over the course of their lifetime. As a result, most people are not fully expressing all of who they truly are. There is no freedom in that way of life. It is stifling, controlling and always puts individuals on danger alert. As a result, it causes people to look and feel constricted and old.

So How Can I Fully Express All of My Emotions,
Be Free and Look Radiant?

The first step is to recognize the presence of a negative emotion. Many people are so unconscious that they don't even know that negative emotions are running them until those emotions jump up and bite them on their bottom at the most inconvenient times.

Ever have the experience of going about your day, minding your own business and then out of the blue, someone says something that triggers your suppressed negative emotions and you unexpectedly lash out? You are as shocked as the person on the receiving end of this inappropriate outburst. Once you can recognize that the negative emotions are present, you can begin to apply the tools and exercises in this chapter to release them.

When you funnel down every emotion, there is only love, and the absence of love, which is fear. Take rage for example. Underneath the rage is anger, underneath the anger is hurt and underneath the hurt is fear. The same thing holds true for prejudice, envy and all other low vibration feelings. Fear is at the core of all of these negative emotions.

As you clear the fear, you give yourself permission to feel your anger, rage, guilt, shame, pain, etc. This is a wonderful gift and it is incredibly freeing and healing. It is important to remember that you can have your feelings without throwing them onto someone else.

As you do this clearing work, you'll discover that your ability to express your innate joy, love, enthusiasm, passion and generosity increases exponentially. Before you know it, you're radiating from the inside out.

Becoming Undeniable

As your divine qualities continue to rise to the surface and freely express, you'll notice that you're becoming absolutely undeniable to everyone. People gravitate to you; they want to be around you and in your lovely energy field. The more you clear the fear, the more your joy and love overflow and the more alluring and attractive you become.

This resulting radiance is the source of everything you most deeply wish to manifest from your divine employment, to an intimate relationship and from deeper richer friendships, to better health and wellness. Every area of your life expands as a result of cultivating this radiance through the release of toxic emotions.

Forgive for the Sheer Vanity of it

When you hang on to old feelings of anger and bitterness, it only hurts you. Holding onto resentment of others is like drinking rat poison and expecting the other person to die. Forgiving is like a facelift for the soul. It also does wonders for the body.

The Power of Vulnerability and the Pain of Shame

"VULNERABILITY IS THE KEY TO REAL INTIMATE MEANINGFUL RELATIONSHIPS. IT IS THE BIRTH PLACE OF JOY, CREATIVITY, BELONGING AND LOVE."

–Dr. Brené Brown, Vulnerability Expert and author of "Daring Greatly"

Recently I was introduced to the work of Dr. Brené Brown, author of several best selling books including, "Daring Greatly" on Oprah Winfrey's Channel. Brené's work offers a new and empowering look at the gifts of being vulnerable.

My interest in including it here is that when you can embrace vulnerability, release shame and guilt, you will experience incredible joy and love. The byproducts of these actions are extraordinary radiance and youthfulness.

"SHAME IS LETHAL. PUT SHAME IN A PETRI DISH, ADD SECRECY, SILENCE AND JUDGMENT AND IT WILL GROW EXPONENTIALLY, IT WILL CREEP INTO EVERY CREVICE AND CORNER OF YOUR LIFE. DOUSE SHAME WITH EMPATHY AND YOU CREATE AN ENVIRONMENT THAT IS HOSTILE TO SHAME. SHAME CAN NOT SURVIVE BEING SPOKEN."
–Dr. Brené Brown, Vulnerability Expert and author of "Daring Greatly"

If you feel uncomfortable reading this section on shame and vulnerability, I highly recommend picking up Brené's books and give yourself the gift of exposing shame to the light of day so you can release it. Shame keeps you separate from the two things that human beings want most, to be loved and to belong. The freedom you will experience from stepping into your authentic vulnerability will not only shower your life with love and joy, it will naturally make you look 15-20 years younger.

Toxic Relationships

As you begin to release what no longer serves you, you start to see clearly which relationships support you and which take away from you.

It may be time to give your relationships a thorough spring-cleaning. The one thing I have discovered over the years is that when I let go of relationships that are no longer mutually supportive and loving, what shows up for me are relationships that are even more loving and supportive. It's always an upgrade… every time.

Exercise #5 Relationship Evaluation Exercise

- Take a minute and make a list of the important relationships in your life.
- Close your eyes and place your focus on your breath for a couple of minutes to get centered and relaxed.
- Now open your eyes, go down that list and ask your body how it feels when you bring this person to mind. Does your body relax and feel good or do you tense up and feel stressed.
- You may be surprised at how your body reacts. This is an especially powerful exercise to do with people you are dating. Our bodies don't lie. Even if you are really into that person, if your body tenses up, it's telling you something.
- If your body does tense up as you think of this person, ask yourself, "Why did we cross paths? What is the gift of this person's presence in my life?" It may be a life lesson or an opportunity to release an old wound or behavioral pattern this person triggers in you.
- If it's not serving you, say thank you for the gift or lesson this relationship gave you, bless it and let it go in love.
- Love, relationship and communications expert, Alison Armstrong speaks of dating as an opportunity to sort. There are millions of available men and women in the world. There is no scarcity when it comes to dating. Only scarcity consciousness keeps you in a relationship that is not serving you. If it's not a great fit, move on. There are plenty of other fish in the sea.

Feng Shui

Clearing and cleaning out your physical spaces, i.e. your home and work surroundings, is also a very important part of detoxing.

Feng Shui is the ancient art of allowing the energies to flow in your environment. This is very important to your overall health, wellbeing and prosperity. Each area of your home and office space pertains to specific dimensions of your life. (See Feng Shui Map Next Page)

Clutter blocks the natural flow of energy in your space. The clearer and cleaner the energy, the more balanced you'll feel and the greater ease you'll have in manifesting what you want in your life.

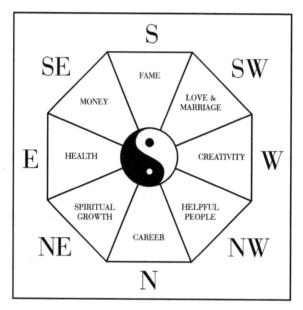

Use this map as a guide to help you incorporate the practice of Feng Shui in your life.

Tips for clearing out your space:

- Make sure to open up your doors and windows when you clear your space. A lot of energy gets circulated when you clean and it's important to release it.
- Keep your living space clean and clutter free.
- Even if you live in small quarters, always allocate a place for every thing and then always put it back in its place. This helps you keep your living area clean, clear and clutter free.
- An orderly environment allows the mind and energy to flow much more freely and lends itself to a greater expression of creativity.
- Make a habit of clearing out regularly. Clutter and junk have a way of piling up quickly. At the first sign of a mess, clean it up immedi-

ately. You'll feel much better and be much more productive in a clean environment.

Taking the Mystery and Mystique out of Meditation

Now that you have begun to clear out what no longer serves you, physically, mentally, emotionally and in your relationships, it's time to give you some tools and exercises to help you maintain the sense of peace, calm and well being that detoxing brings. One of the simplest ways to do this is meditation.

What is meditation and why is it so significant to your health and wellbeing? How does it contribute to your radiance and youthfulness?

There are a lot of misconceptions about meditation. The word can conjure up images of a yogi wrapped up like a pretzel sitting on a bed of nails. It is actually a very straightforward process.

"PRAYER IS HOW YOU TALK TO GOD... MEDITATION IS HOW GOD TALKS TO YOU."
–Deepak Chopra, Spiritual Teacher, Physician and Best Selling Author

Simply put, meditation is how Spirit speaks to you. It can help you with everything from manifesting abundance to creating greater health and peace of mind. It is also beneficial for dealing with the daily stresses of life. Meditation helps quiet your mind so that you can tap into the infinite wisdom of the Universe.

"LIKE A RADIO STATION, KGOD IS BROADCASTING 24/7/365... ALL YOU HAVE TO DO IS QUIET THE MIND TO TUNE INTO THIS FREQUENCY."
–Dr. Michael Beckwith, Spiritual Teacher and Author of "Spiritual Liberation"

When you meditate not only do you relieve stress, you actually stop the aging process. That's right. Each time you step into meditation you are literally turning back the hands of time. Talk about having access to the fountain of youth at your fingertips.

Types of Meditations

There's no need to be intimidated by meditation. There are many different types of meditation, and it is easy to find one that works for you.

Here's a list of some common meditations:

- Moving Meditations
- Walking Meditations
- Exercise Meditations
- Singing Meditations
- Dancing Meditations
- Music Meditations
- Laughing Meditations
- Guided Meditations
- Making Love (Tantra)

There are some wonderful books and CDs on meditation. I have listed a few of them in the reference section of this book which is located on my website, www.DrElizabeth.com.

Meditation Exercise

Here's a simple meditation exercise that you can do anytime you want to feel more peaceful and grounded. It is great if you can meditate for 10 minutes or more, but even 30 seconds or a minute can do wonders to center you.

Sit in a quiet and comfortable place where you will not be disturbed. Place your feet firmly on the ground and gently close your eyes. Take several long slow deep yoga breaths. Place your right hand on your stomach. Expand your ribcage and allow your abdominal muscles to push your hand out as you inhale. This allows your diaphragm to expand so that you can fill your entire lung cavity with air. Relax your shoulders on the in breath. Push your stomach in as you exhale. Repeat. Place your left hand on your heart. This allows you to connect with the energy of Universal love.

If your mind begins to wander, place your attention on your breath. Follow it into your body as you inhale. See it circulating and bringing renewed energy and vitality. Then watch the old energy release out of your body as you exhale.

Awareness is the First Clue

Meditation can be very helpful during stressful times and can be done almost anywhere at anytime. The key to successfully using meditation during stressful situations is awareness. Begin to hone that light bulb of perception that says, "Oh yes, I'm experiencing stress in my body right now. It's time for me to regain my balance."

One day I found myself losing my center at a very important business meeting. I noticed I was becoming fearful. I felt a sharp pain in my gut and my breathing became shallow and rapid.

You Can Always Go to the Bathroom

Once I recognized that I was experiencing fear, I quickly excused myself from the meeting and went to the ladies room. I sat down on the commode, took a couple of long, slow, deep breaths and began to quiet my mind. Within a matter of minutes, the fear dissipated. I returned to the conference room, refreshed and reconnected to my higher self. Just that short visit to the rest room shifted my entire energy and outcome of the meeting for the better. The next time you find yourself in a stressful situation, I invite you to try this simple technique.

Guided Meditations

If you are new to this sacred practice, or if you are just having difficulty with it, I highly recommend guided meditations. In these meditations, a teacher uses his or her voice to gently guide you into a meditative state. Many guided meditations incorporate theta healing music, which allows the listener to gracefully and easily slip into a peaceful and relaxed state for maximum benefits.

Theta Music Healing

There are days when life's challenges can really take their toll on me. One of the most powerful and effective tools I have discovered to alleviate stress is theta healing music meditations.

What is a theta healing music meditation, and how does it work?

Theta is that magical brainwave state experienced in dreams, just before falling asleep and just upon waking. Theta brain waves have the ability to help access the subconscious and therefore are powerful tools for healing. Many important messages can be received in this peaceful state.

Theta healing music puts you into a deep theta brainwave configuration, allowing you to attain a richer state of relaxation and a more profound meditation. The benefits of this include improved sleep, increased levels of peacefulness and stress reduction.

Intuitive Intelligence and Energetic Healing

Now that you have been introduced to meditation, I'd like to familiarize you with another powerful healing modality that has been incredibly beneficial in my own life, intuitive intelligence.

I learned about intuitive intelligence healing years ago and I have seen first hand in my own life and in the lives of countless others, the profound results that this healing modality provides.

What is Intuitive Intelligence?

Intuitive intelligence is a form of energetic healing, otherwise known as clairvoyant or psychic healing.

There are tremendous misconceptions and fears around the words psychic, clairvoyant and intuition. All those late night advertisements for the psychic hotline just add fuel to the fire.

When some people hear the word psychic or clairvoyant, it conjures up images of a charlatan sitting in front of a crystal ball in a dark room asking for money to tell them their future. The true meaning of these words is far different than most people assume.

Merriam-Webster Dictionary defines Psychic as, "Of or pertaining to the human soul or mind, spiritual". Now, that doesn't sound very "woo-woo" or scary at all.

My clairvoyant teacher and healer, Vicki Reiner, defines the word psychic as "of the soul." She also uses the words intuitive intelligence to describe her work. I appreciate this phrase because it lands safely on most people's ears when they hear it. It also perfectly describes what clairvoyance and psychic abilities actually are.

Owning Your Intuitive Intelligence

Many people mistakenly assume that only a select few possess psychic abilities. However, the truth is that everyone is born with the gift of intuition, psychic abilities and clairvoyance, which is defined as "clear seeing." It comes standard with every human body. This intuition is a form of intelligence that is available to all of us anytime we wish to access it.

As a child, I was having spiritual thoughts and experiences at a very early age. I often knew things before they happened. I have always had a profound sense of unconditional love and a tremendous capacity to share that love with others, even strangers. In addition, I have a deep sense of connection to others and an innate awareness that kindness, compassion, love and joy are always the answers to any question or challenge.

When I was in kindergarten, I remember thinking, if only people could see the "inside" of another person, then they would be able to see their true beauty. Being raised strict catholic and having to go to church on a daily basis, I somehow knew at a very early age that religions separate and spirituality and unconditional love unites.

I recall leaving my body and traveling often from a very early age. I also came into this lifetime knowing how to warp time and drop into the abyss of the Universe. At the time, however, I had no idea what it was I was doing. I just did it naturally.

I remember, as a child, going into my parent's bedroom one particular night wanting to explain my spiritual adventures. My mother just looked at me sideways and tucked me under her arm. There are days she still looks at me sideways.

Many of you had similar spiritual experiences. You may have had "imaginary friends." Maybe you could hear what people were thinking or knew what was going to happen before it occurred. These experiences can be very frightening, disturbing and isolating. Therefore, people often turn off their powerful and empowering clairvoyant gifts.

You might have tried to explain your experiences to your family and friends, resulting in ridicule, or you just kept them to yourself out of fear of being mocked or considered different or odd.

Either way, many of you suppressed these wonderful and powerful gifts that reside in you. Even if you don't remember having a specific intuitive experience growing up, the gift is still there inside you waiting to be accessed. Now is the time to awaken and embrace these gifts and begin to incorporate them back into your daily life.

Many people desire to access their intuition again and ask me how to do this. Here's an easy exercise to help you ground and tap into your own intuitive intelligence:

Chakras

A simple awareness of the main chakras of the body is necessary in doing this exercise. Chakras are wheels of light, life force energy, found within the body. There are seven major chakras in the body. In addition there are numerous other chakras in various locations throughout the body including the hands and the feet. There are also chakras that extend several feet above the crown of the head. Clearing the chakras is a great way to release negative energy.

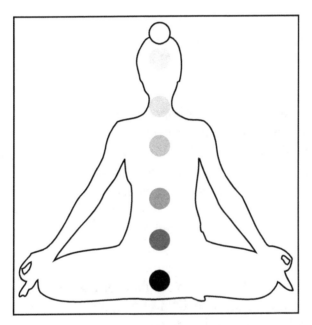

Diagram of the 7 major chakras of the body

"Grounding Cord Meditation"

Find a place where you can sit quietly and not be interrupted for 10 minutes. Place your feet on the floor and your back against the chair. Place your right hand on your tummy and your left hand on your heart.

Close your eyes and begin to relax. Start observing your breath as it enters your body and leaves again. Relax your shoulders and allow your diaphragm to drop and your rib cage expand with every in breath. As you take in the air, your tummy and ribcage should expand outward. To assist you with your breathing, imagine that you are pushing your hand that is resting on your tummy out with each in breath. As you expire the air, contract your diaphragm, rib cage and abdominal muscles. One clue to let you know that you are doing this breath correctly is that you will feel the hand that is resting on your stomach move out as you inhale and in as you exhale. This is the breath used when practicing yoga and meditation.

If you need further assistance or would like more guidance on this practice, I offer a "Sacred Yoga/Meditation Breath" CD on my website, www. DrElizabeth.com

Now continue to breathe slowly and deeply. Place your attention and your energy in your 6th chakra, in the center of your head. Light it up with a starburst of light. You can use the image of fireworks exploding in the night sky. This starburst technique is used as a way to say hello to each chakra and activate it. Feel your entire being sitting inside this powerful chakra. From your 6th chakra, look down (from inside your body) at your 1st chakra, located at the base of your spine, and again, light it up with a starburst of light.

From the bottom of your 1st chakra, extend a cord all the way down into the middle of Mother Earth. You can see this cord as a beam of light, a tree trunk, a string of pearls, a steal beam, a waterfall or whatever image works for you. This is called your grounding cord.

Once that cord/beam is firmly planted into the earth, observe how your body feels. Do you feel more grounded, centered, calm and/or peaceful? Many people experience these feelings when they place their grounding cord firmly into Mother Earth.

Now with your attention and energy still in your 6th chakra, picture a chain with a handle attached to it directly in front of you. (Imagine one of those old fashioned toilets with a chain that you pull to flush.) You can also use the image of a big red button. In your mind's eye, reach up and pull the chain or push the red button. As you do, ask your body to release any feelings of fear that you are ready to let go of now. You can actually see and feel the energy of fear releasing from your body and traveling down the grounding cord. Sometimes the energy can look like waves or lines flowing out of your body. Do not worry about sending the energy of fear into Mother Earth. She is powerful beyond our comprehension and has the capacity to take all the negative energy that you release and transmute and transform it into beautiful loving energy. So release away.

As you begin to release the energy of fear, notice how it makes your body feel. You may feel lighter, calmer, more peaceful and joyous. You may also have the sense that you have more "room" in your body. This is because you are releasing energy that does not belong to you.

Next I invite you to release the energy of doubt and worry. Reach up, pull the chain or push the big red button and let whatever energy of doubt and worry that is present in your body release.

This time you are going to release anger. As you pull the chain or push the red button, feel the energy of anger leaving your body and flowing down your grounding cord into Mother Earth.

Take as much time as you'd like to let go of whatever negative energies your body is ready to release.

Continue to hold your attention and energy in your 6th chakra, in the center of your head. From this space, look up at the top of your head. This is your 7th chakra. See the peaceful, neutral Cosmic energy from Father Universe streaming into you from the top of your head. As you are doing this, continue breathing slowly and deeply. Let the energy flow in from the top of your head and fill your entire body with this beautiful energy.

Next, with your feet still planted firmly on the floor, open up your feet chakras, located at the balls of your feet. Allow the healing neutral energy of Mother Earth to flow up through your feet, up your legs and into your body. Then send it down the grounding cord.

When I first started doing this practice, I wondered why it was important to bring "neutral" energy into the body. I assumed that positive energy would be a better choice. However, my clairvoyant teacher, Vicki Reiner taught me the importance of getting neutral to a particular energy, person or situation before we can release it. Once we achieve neutrality, we can easily and effortlessly clear negativity out of our physical and energetic space.

Once you have released all the negative energy your body is ready to clear at this time, imagine a beautiful, big, bright, glowing sun over your head. Fill that sun with all of your beautiful sparkling energy. Place your joy, your dreams, your wishes, your desires, your energy and your light into that radiant shining ball of sunlight. When you have completed filling your golden sun with your energy, reach up with both of your hands and grab hold of your sun and pour it into your body through the top of your head.

See and feel that glowing golden liquid light pouring into your body. Fill in all of those places where you released the negative energies of fear, anger, doubt, etc., with this beautiful liquid sunlight. This is your energy. It is the essence of who you really are. Take slow deep breaths and see and feel your energy filling up your entire body and flowing all the way down your grounding cord.

Once you have completed this, slowly open your eyes and come back into the room. Feel the peace, calm and relaxation filling your entire being.

You can do this exercise as often as you wish. I recommend doing it once a day or anytime you're experiencing low vibration energy, such as anger, fear or doubt.

NOTE: this exercise allows you to release a tremendous amount of negative energy. You may feel sleepy or light headed during or after this exercise. You may also feel heavy or "unconscious." This is the unwanted energy that does not belong to you, leaving your body. You may also feel quite light, peaceful and high once you've completed this exercise. Getting rid of heavy energy that is not yours can feel wonderful. Whatever you feel is okay. Utilize this exercise as often as possible for maximum detoxification and clearing. Make sure you drink plenty of purified water and get lots of rest when practicing this clearing technique.

Science has proven that we are all made up of energy. One of the challenges we unknowingly face is the existence of other people's energy in our space. This can cause all sorts of difficulties physically, emotionally and mentally. I was shocked to discover that the negative energy causing me so much pain in my life was not even mine.

The good news is that once you are aware of this fact, you can clear it out. In my work with Vicki, I have been able to eliminate an enormous amount of negative energy. The results have been more creativity, joy, freedom and the manifestation of this book.

This practice is a powerful clearing tool to release the unwelcome energy of others in your life. It is also a wonderful emotional and mental detoxification exercise. I invite you to give it a try. It is one of the simplest and quickest methods for removing negative energy and the results are tremendous peace, a wonderful sense of wellbeing and a radiant youthful glow.

This practice was inspired by and based on the teachings of Vicki Reiner and the practice of meditation.

The Power of Intuitive Intelligence

Most people, when faced with a challenging decision, look outside themselves for the answer. This can be very dangerous and disempowering. The truth is you always know what is best for you. However, when you are not tuned into your intuitive intelligence, it's difficult to see the right answer. A noisy mind can never "see" clearly. When people get scared and reach outside themselves for their answers, often times the guidance that is given is inaccurate, inappropriate and not in their best interest.

The benefits of owning your own clairvoyance are numerous. It gives you the ability to make wise decisions. This in turn allows you to stand in your own power. It is very empowering to be able to wisely navigate life's difficult choices on your own. Not to say you can't turn to someone else who also is dialed into their intuitive intelligence to give you guidance. However, when you already own your own clear seeing, it is easier to know whom to turn to for rich and empowering guidance. When you're open, available and already dialed into the intuitive intelligence field, another word for the Divine Universe, you are led to profound and tremendously synchronistic guidance. Here's an example from my own life.

1994 was a particularly challenging time for me. My beloved maternal grandfather, whom I adored, made his transition (another word for saying he passed away). In addition, a long-term relationship I was involved in came to an abrupt conclusion. I went from living in a beautiful home over-looking the ocean in Santa Barbara to living with two girls whom I didn't know very well in a small apartment in Los Angeles. I felt very alone in the world and very unsure of myself and my future.

One weekday afternoon I was on my way to a life enhancement class when I remembered that I left my journal at home. I parked my car in the driveway, locked it and quickly ran upstairs to my apartment to retrieve my journal. Since I was just dashing up to my apartment for a minute, I left my purse and bag sitting on the passenger seat of my locked car. In the amount of time it took me to run up, grab my journal and return to my car, someone had smashed the passenger side window of my car and removed both my bag and my purse. As is true for many women, my entire life was in those two satchels.

I was just about to embark on a mental tirade of, "Really? Why did this have to happen to me? As if my life doesn't suck enough, now I have a busted car window and my most important possessions are gone." But instead, I took a very long, slow, deep breath and in that moment, a miracle occurred.

That breath pre-empted the mental diatribe and calmed me down just long enough to hear the voice of Spirit whisper in my ear, "Go to your sister's home and cancel your credit cards."

One of my younger sisters, Suzanne lived about a mile away and I happened to have the clicker to her underground parking garage. I realized that my car would be safe there while I used her home phone (this was long before the arrival of cell phones) to call and report my stolen credit cards.

As I stopped at a four way stop sign, then proceeded to cross through the intersection, I heard the voice say, "Turn around, drive down the alley way and look in the garage bin." Now I had heard the voice of Spirit, (call it what you want, your higher self, God, the Universe, your inner knowing, whatever works for you) many times throughout the course of my life. And yet, the clarity and surety of this message astounded me.

I literally began a conversation with this voice saying, "Really? You want me to turn around, drive down an alley, open up a garbage bin and expect to find my possessions?" But something in me, greater than my inner skeptic gently but firmly grabbed hold of my thoughts and my steering wheel and in that moment, I pulled a U-turn right in the middle of the intersection and drove my car down the alley. I parked in front of the garbage container and slowly opened up the lid. Much to my astonishment, there was my bag, with all my precious possessions still inside.

Immediately, after saying, "Thank you," I began to rifle through the other garbage bins near by looking for my purse. My logical mind assessed that if my bag was here, my purse had to be somewhere in the local vicinity. But the voice softly said, "Your purse is not here Sweetheart. Go to your sister's home and cancel your credit cards."

Not to argue with the same voice that miraculously guided me to my bag, I quickly placed the lids back down on the garbage bins in gratitude and drove uneventfully to my sister's home.

After canceling my credit cards, I sat down on the couch, took another long, slow, deep breath and patiently awaited further instructions. I didn't have to wait long. The voice ensued, "Go back to your home right now." So I hopped in my car and drove back to my apartment.

No sooner did I park my car, I saw a uniformed police officer half way down the street walking towards my apartment. He was holding a large black hefty garbage bag in his hand. The voice said, "He's got your purse." I walked over to him and said, "You have my handbag don't you?"

He was shocked. He knew who I was from my driver's license photo, but he couldn't figure out how in the world I knew that he was in possession of my purse.

When Spirit guides you, which it is continuously doing, It always gives you comprehensive instructions. Your inner wisdom will let you know who to tell what information and when it is suitable to share it. It will also tell you when it is not appropriate to say something because that person would not have the capacity to understand. When the policeman asked me how I knew that he had my purse, Spirit whispered, "It's not appropriate to share" and I just said, "Lucky guess," smiled, gave him a big hug and said thank you. This is just one example of the powerful guidance available to you and me all the time.

Time and time again, I will hear my inner voice whisper to me, "Tell this person that they look beautiful today," or "Let this person know that everything's going to be okay." The messages given to me are always very specific and often times include information that I would not otherwise be privy to having.

These invitations to share information with people began when I was quite young. At first I'd say, "Really? You want me to walk up to this total stranger and tell them…that?" However, what began happening was that these people would inevitably say, "How did you know that I needed to hear that today?" Or, "Thank you so much for saying that, you made my day!"

It is absolutely astonishing each time Spirit whispers a message in my ear for someone, the person lights up with appreciation and gratitude when I deliver it. It never fails. I'm pretty accustomed to this, but every once in a while even I will ask, "Really, you want me to tell them that?" Never once have I been led astray. And, each one of you has that ability as well.

"EVERYWHERE YOU GO, YOU'RE GOING TO HAVE THE OPPORTUNITY TO TOUCH SOME-ONE'S LIFE SO ALWAYS MAKE IT FOR THE BETTER."
–*Lucille Rochetta Inda (Dr Elizabeth's Mom) Registered Nurse and Mother Extraordinaire*

Most of the time we have no idea how we impact the lives of the people who cross our path on a daily basis. Just a smile or a kind word can make an extraordinary difference in someone's life. We know this but in the hustle and bustle of our everyday lives, we often forget to take advantage of these beautiful opportunities to share our hearts with others.

Here's a powerful story that demonstrates the importance of always being aware of the chance to share our love with others in simple and yet profound ways.

To Honk or Not to Honk… That is the Question

I'll never forget this particular story shared by Dr. Caroline Myss. It touched my heart so deeply that it made me cry and I often share it when I speak at conferences. It serves as a constant reminder to me of the power of love, grace and prayer.

A woman who attended one of Caroline's seminars shared this story of her near death experience. This woman was in a terrible car accident. It was so severe that she had already left her body by the time the paramedics were placing her in the ambulance.

Once out of her body, she was immediately raised out of the 3rd dimension physical realm. From this elevated awareness she could clearly hear all the thoughts of the people in the other cars. Some were profoundly shaken; others were honking their horn, annoyed by the delay caused by the accident.

Suddenly she felt this overwhelming sense of light and love emanating from one of the cars. As she realized that this particular driver was offering her prayers, she was transported directly to the car. In her non-physical state, the injured woman easily memorized the license plate of the individual who was offering her these sweet prayers.

The woman in the car accident was in a coma for weeks and had an arduous recovery, but she never forgot the woman who prayed for her. Once fully recuperated, she tracked down the woman via her license plate, went to her home with a bouquet of flowers and said, "Do you remember that terrible car accident several months back? You were praying for the person in that car." The woman acknowledged that she did remember that incident. "I was the person in that accident and your sweet prayers made an enormous difference during that experience and in my recovery. Thank You."

This is not an isolated or random incident. Every day, each one of us has the opportunity to shine our light and love on others and make a profound difference in their lives. Unlike the woman in this story, we may never know what difference our light, love and prayers make. But have no doubt; each act of kindness, every smile and loving word touches the heart and soul of the person on the receiving end of our grace filled actions.

Sometimes when I'm rushing around town, I like to remind myself of that story. It always inspires me to pause and ask the question, "How can I bless those around me today?" That reminder can be the difference between honking and blessing.

A Birthday Gift that Changed My Life Forever

When I turned 50, I was happy being a journalist. I caught a powerful vision to share the wisdom of teachers around the world as a talk show host. I co-hosted a nationally syndicated talk show and loved it. In addition, I had just completed a series of interviews of inspiring people who were making a difference with their messages. I loved the idea of using the media to bring uplifting content to a world that is hungry for it.

My dear friend Kelly gifted me with a clairvoyant reading from her colleague and close friend, Diana as a 50th birthday gift. The very first thing this talented reader said was, "You're a speaker and you're going to be sharing your message on very large stages within six months."

Even though Kelly, who is also powerfully intuitive, had been telling me this fact for months and I had spoken on stages giving passionate and inspirational talks since I was in grade school, I felt myself go into major resistance. I heard myself begin to say, "No, no, no... I'm not a speaker." But then remembered my experience ten years ago, when a clairvoyant reminded me that I was a dancer. So, I reluctantly surrendered and simply listened.

I was astonished to hear this information. Enormous amounts of energy began flowing through me. My mind was racing with all of these thoughts, "I'm an interviewer, not a speaker... I interview speakers. What in the world would I even talk about?"

Even as my mind was spinning and I was fighting this concept, there was something much deeper and greater in me that was beginning to awaken to what Diana was sharing. I countered my resistance with slow, deep breaths and relaxation techniques. I surrendered to the Divine message that was coming through this wonderful intuitive reader.

As I continued to breathe and ground, this energy of excitement began to emerge from the very core of my being. My hands were on fire. Energy was pulsing through me at warp speed, lighting up my entire being with the most radiant and beautiful energy. It was more intense than anything I'd ever experienced in my life.

As I fully embraced her words, I began to catch this magnificent vision that she was sharing with me. In this state of surrender, I was able to "grasp" with my 6th chakra what she was "seeing" through her own 6th chakra and hear the Divine whispers that she was listening to.

Sure enough, six months to the date of my reading, I found myself on stage at an international conference speaking to a very large audience. And, just as Diana had predicted, my message revealed itself to me joyfully, easily and effortlessly.

"ONCE IN A GREAT WHILE WE ARE OFFERED A VIEW FROM THE MOUNTAINTOP AND THEN WE ARE TRANSPORTED BACK TO THE FLOOR OF THE FOREST. IT IS THAT VIEW FROM THE MOUNTAINTOP THAT CARRIES US THROUGH OUR DAY TO DAY EXISTENCE."
–Marianne Williamson, Spiritual Teacher and Best Selling Author

I share this story with you because it demonstrates the power that clairvoyant readings and healings can provide. Some days we live our lives on the mountaintop and other times we are in the midst of the wilderness. Readings provide clarity, guidance and encouragement at times when we may not be able to see the forest through the trees.

I was just hoping to be an interviewer, but the reading offered me a glimpse of a life and profession that was greater than I could have ever dreamed possible. I was shown a career that included sharing my own message and interviewing others as well. It was absolutely perfect for me.

In addition, at this point in my life I had already owned my own intuitive intelligence. Therefore I was able to recognize the guidance that was being channeled through this particular reader on my behalf as poignant and invaluable.

The other reason I share this story with you is to demonstrate the tremendous value of clairvoyant/intuitive readings when approached from an open mind and a healthy emotional and mental state.

The Healing Benefits of Readings

Clairvoyant readings offer more than just a glimpse into our future. They offer a powerful and effective method of healing and clearing as well as tremendous insight and guidance. These readings can help you release old energy and toxins that have been stored in the body for years, sometimes lifetimes.

The important thing is to approach the healing with the awareness that significant clearing can occur when you actively participate in the healing and you are ready and willing to release that which no longer serves you on your soul's evolutionary path.

I am truly blessed to have extraordinarily gifted intuitives, clairvoyants, healers and energy workers in my life. Their expertise affords me avenues to continuously heal and clear. The peace, joy, freedom and clarity I have garnered from these techniques have been life enhancing. I offer these healings as a tool to assist you in your own journey as well.

In the reference section of this book, which you can find on my website, www.DrElizabeth.com, I offer a list of clairvoyants and healers I have had the pleasure to work with. They are all brilliant and talented and I invite you to check out their services.

Dream Healing

"OUR DREAMS ARE LIKE GOLD, THEY ARE OUR GREATEST ALLY IN LIFE AND ALSO THE THING WE MOST TAKE FOR GRANTED."
–Kelly Sullivan Walden, Dream Expert and Author of "I Had the Strangest Dream"

It is scientifically proven that we all dream three to nine times a night.

However, most people do not even remember their dreams. Our dreams are a rich source of guidance and tremendous healing.

In western society, where people rush around from the moment they awake until the moment they plop down onto their beds utterly exhausted, dreams do not hold a high priority. However, indigenous cultures around the world know the incredible value of messages mined from the dream realm.

Dreams are Spirit and your subconscious speaking to you. If you will begin to court your night time dreams like a lover, they will reveal rich secrets that can help you manifest your daytime desires.

A very dear friend and colleague of mine, dream expert, Kelly Sullivan Walden wrote several wonderful books on the subject of dreams, including "I Had the Strangest Dream…the Dreamer's Dictionary for the 21st Century," and "It's All in Your Dreams." These books explain in great detail how to remember your dreams and interpret their rich and life enhancing messages. I highly recommend picking up a copy and keeping it on your nightstand.

In the meantime, here are some simple and easy techniques Kelly suggests to remember your dreams.

Exercise #6 How to Remember Your Dreams

- Declare that you will remember your dreams before you go to sleep.
- Place something to record your dreams on your nightstand.
- If possible, wake up naturally instead of using an alarm.
- As soon as you awake, before going over what you need to do for the day or jumping out of bed, lay there for a minute and allow your dreams to reveal themselves to you.
- Even a tiny little piece of a dream is like a golden thread that can lead you back to the entire reverie.
- Take a question or idea you have been pondering with you into your sleepy time and ask for your dreams to give you an answer.

The Power of Dreams

Many incredible messages can come through dreams, I know this first-hand because I was the recipient of one of those extraordinary messages.

While I was writing this book, Kelly called me one morning in a flurry of excitement and proclaimed, "I had a dream about you last night!" Now, when anyone has a dream about you, it's always a gift, but when world-class dream expert, Kelly Sullivan Walden calls you up and says, "I had a dream about you," you know it's going to be something extraordinary… and, it was.

Kelly knew that I had been toying around with various titles for my upcoming book. When she called me that morning I never imagined that she was gifting me with the title of my book, "Skinny Dipping in the Fountain of Youth."

One of the many extraordinary things about swimming in the fountain of youth is that synchronicities become common occurrences. When she told me the name, I was in awe and overcome with gratitude and delight. I absolutely adore this title and the fact that it came directly from the Universe through my amazing friend, Kelly in a dream, makes it even more special and delicious.

If I can be gifted the title of my book through a dream, imagine what is possible for you. Let me know what life-enhancing messages come to you through your dreams. I can't wait to hear all about them.

Sweet Dreams

While we're on the subject of dreams, I'd like to say just a word or two about sleep. For anyone over the age of thirty five, especially women, sleep is your best friend. And for those of you men and women who are over forty, I invite you to embrace this health benefit with wild abandon. Your body will love you for it.

"Juicy Sleep"

Not only is it important to get eight hours of sleep, when you get that sleep is equally important. The sleep you get between 10pm and midnight is incredibly nourishing. This is when the body replenishes those juicy hormones that help you look and feel your most sexy, youthful, beautiful self. I call this particular sleep, "Juicy Sleep" because of its incredibly rejuvenating and youth promoting benefits.

This can be quite discouraging especially for all you die-hard night owls. Being a self proclaimed night owl myself for years, once I embraced my 10pm bedtime, I couldn't refute the significant benefits I was seeing and feeling in my face and body.

Tips for getting your sexy sleep on:

- Plan to get 8 hours of sleep a night. Schedule it into your calendar if necessary.
- The goal is to be asleep by 10pm (I know, I know, this is a tough one for those of you with a lively social life).
- Turn off the computer and/or TV around 9pm.
- Take a nice relaxing bath around 9:15-9:30pm.
- Light some candles, turn on some soothing music and just enjoy.
- Those of you with kids, and/or lots of evening responsibilities, don't worry if you can only spare a couple of minutes, a 3 minute bath will go a long way towards helping you unwind and get ready for bed. It's also a wonderful gift of self-love.
- Crawl into bed by about 9:45pm and either read or do a little meditation
- Turn the lights off by 10pm.
- Set your alarm for 6am (even if you don't have to get up this early) what this does is reset your body clock and sleep schedule.
- You can use that extra time for a beautiful morning meditation, journaling, yoga, exercising or just catching up on some reading, work or other activities.

NOTE to diehard night owls: Anyone can shift their sleep schedule. If you want to reap the incredibly rich youthing benefits of "Juicy Sleep," give this technique a try. You'll be so grateful that you did and your face will thank you for it.

Healing Modalities that Fly Just Under the Radar

There is a multitude of healing modalities available today that are far less familiar to the general population. I refer to these techniques as healing modalities that fly just under the radar. I feel that it's important for people to know that they have a myriad of options when dealing with their personal health and wellbeing.

Here's a list of some of these powerful techniques:

- Acupuncture
- Bodywork
- Energetic healing
- Energy medicine
- Pranic healing
- Light and radio frequency healing
- Quantum healing
- Sound healing with crystal bowls, drums and other musical instruments
- Numerology
- Astrology
- Tarot cards
- Angel readings
- Swimming with the dolphins
- Watsu

Being open to the information that is available through these various alternative modalities can offer relief from physical, emotional and mental suffering as well as provide you with wonderful information and guidance.

See the reference section of the book located on my website DrElizabeth. com for a list of recommended practitioners.

"The Menopause Monster"

NOTE: to my readers in their twenties and thirties. Although menopause doesn't apply to you directly at this stage in your life, I invite you to read this section of the book. You may have a parent or relative who is struggling with "The Menopause Monster" and this information could help them circumvent this challenge. Trust me, they will be eternally grateful to you.

Many people from around the world have contacted me asking for assistance in dealing with menopause. Since this is a subject I know about from experience, I wanted to share what I learned through my own journey into menopause and my subsequent "healing" from this very challenging condition.

"The Menopause Monster," as I affectionately call this phase, is a very trying time in a woman or man's life. Many people are not well informed about the changes that may occur in their body. It is different for everyone; however, I want people to know that now there are powerful solutions available to you when "The Menopause Monster" strikes.

Part of the challenge of "The Menopause Monster" is that it catches you off guard. One minute you're fine, the next you don't know what hit you. Having gone through menopause and witnessing first hand the ravages it can place on a body, I am deeply passionate about assisting both women and men in counterbalancing the loss of vital sex hormones. One of the keys to conquering "The Menopause Monster" is knowing your options and taking action at the first signs of symptoms.

My Dance with "The Menopause Monster"

"The Menopause Monster" hit me like a ton of bricks. It was as though one day I was completely fine and the next, I didn't even recognize myself.

I looked in the mirror and asked, "Who are you and what did you do with my body?"

I am one of those women who's always taken incredible care of myself. I eat healthy, work out 6 days a week and my physical body has always reflected my commitment to health and wellbeing and my passion for being physically fit.

Then, all of a sudden I began to get hot… really hot, and not in a good way. I was burning up from the inside out. It was the kind of heat that gave me severe nausea and claustrophobia.

I also began noticing other symptoms. I started losing strength and gaining weight, even though I was still eating healthy and exercising diligently. For the first time in my life, I was unable to manage my weight with my healthy lifestyle.

Another unpleasant side effect for me was the appearance of cellulite. Up until this time, cellulite was never an issue for me. After menopause hit, I discovered cellulite in places I didn't even know I could get this unsightly challenge.

I also started waking up in the middle of the night soaking wet, and not because there was a beautiful man next to me.

At my wits end, I reached out to a physician who specializes in Obstetrics and Gynecology, and asked what I could do about this. She replied, unapologetically, "That's just the way it is, kid, you're getting old, get used to it."

I knew in my heart that there was nothing "old" about me. Never being one to take a challenge lying down, I decided that if they can put a man on the moon, there must be something they can do for menopause and I was determined to find someone who was willing to help me.

I asked a friend in the gym who was going through menopause herself what she was doing. She told me enthusiastically that her physician put her on anti depressants for her menopause symptoms. "Are you kidding me?" I thought. I was shocked and appalled. Certainly that was not the solution I was searching for.

So I set out to discover someone who could help restore my physical, mental and emotional states and, in turn, help countless others through my speaking and writing.

Enter Dr. Steven Krems. The arrival of Dr. Krems in my life was very significant. I had made a very strong intention to find a physician, versed in both Western and Eastern medicine, who embraced cutting edge, expansive possibility thinking. After witnessing first hand how he was able to assist a friend of mine, I knew that he was the physician for me.

When I met Dr. Krems, he exceeded my expectations. I shared with him my goals to restore my body back to its pre-menopausal condition and he concurred with an enthusiastic yes. He spent over an hour with me, asking questions and explaining viable options for my symptoms and challenges.

My experience working with Dr. Krems was one of absolute possibility, rooted in feasible and healthy natural solutions. I felt hopeful and grateful to have found him.

"The Sexy Years" by Suzanne Somers

During my first visit, Dr. Krems recommended Suzanne Somers book, "The Sexy Years." I highly suggest reading this book. Suzanne and her team of physicians do a phenomenal job explaining menopause and how to navigate its raging waters safely to sane shores.

My solution to "The Menopause Monster" came, in part, in the form of 100% natural bio identical hormones. These natural hormones don't just mask the symptoms the way their pharmaceutical counterparts do, these bio identical hormones actually replace the sex hormones back into your body.

What that means is your vitality, sexual appetite and juiciness are restored. To a woman like me, that was a Godsend.

Within the first week, my strength began to return. The "hotties," as I affectionately referred to hot flashes, were annihilated, the lethargy subsided and I began to feel like myself again. My sense of youthfulness returned. I had more energy and enthusiasm. To me, these bio identical hormones have been a lifesaver.

There is an enormous amount of data explaining the benefits of bio identical hormone treatment vs. pharmaceutical hormone treatment and also bio identical hormonal treatment vs. no treatment. Speak to a trusted physician or qualified medical professional to make your own decision. Each body is different and each woman and man has to choose for his or herself. For me, going on bio identical hormones was one of the best decisions I ever made.

Male Menopause

Menopause isn't just something that women experience. Men are equally susceptible to the depletion of vital sex hormones and are candidates for all natural bio identical hormonal replacement therapy as well. If you or the man in your life is experiencing a loss in strength, weight gain, depression, fatigue and/or declining libido, natural bio identical hormonal replacement therapy may be the answer.

100% All Natural Skin Treatments for Anti-Aging, Cellulite and Skin Tightening

As I traveled upon my road to recovery from the ravages of "The Menopause Monster," I began to investigate healthy and natural treatments that dealt with my subsequent cellulite and skin elasticity issues. Many people suffer from these conditions. For a long time, there were no cures available. What I learned is that now there is hope for healing these conditions.

I was thrilled to discover that my answer came in the form of 100% all natural cleansing treatments. These new technologies utilize light, sound, radio frequencies and micro-current frequencies to detoxify the body and cleanse the lymphatic system. The added benefit of these cleansing treatments is that they naturally tighten the skin and reduce cellulite. It is a beautiful way to naturally youth yourself from the inside out. Talk about a "Beauty Bonanza."

If you battle with cellulite, sun damage and/or the loss of skin tone and elasticity, regardless of your age or gender, I invite you to check out these remarkable treatments.

I wish I had known about them when I was in the midst of my battle with "The Menopause Monster." One of the things I discovered over the years is that it is so much easier to maintain than it is to restore. If you treat cellulite and the loss of skin elasticity immediately, results are much easier and quicker to achieve and maintain. In other words, don't wait.

If you are in the Los Angeles area, I highly recommend the following salons.

"Per Amore" in Beverly Hills. The name "Per Amore" means, "For love of self" and the owner, Lynn Banfi absolutely lives by this phrase. She offers incredible holistic treatments in a loving and supportive environment.

Other wonderful practitioners offering all natural skin tightening and cellulite treatments are Lori Hart's salon, "About Face and Beyond" in Westwood and Diana Presley in Hollywood.

You can find a list of salons in Los Angeles that offer these treatments in the reference section of this book located on my website, www.DrElizabeth.com.

Natural Products

Other areas to examine for toxicity are the products you use every day. Your skin is the largest organ in your body. Therefore what you put on your body is as important as what you put in it. It's all going to the same place… inside you.

I invite you to look at the ingredients in the products you use everyday. Are there toxins in your toothpaste, your shampoo or your skin cream? If so, there are products on the market that offer non-toxic alternatives.

The next time you visit your health food store, ask for the all-natural skin and hair products section. It's important to be aware of what you're putting on your body for maximum health, radiance and youthfulness.

Once I began detoxing, eating raw and meditating, I noticed that I could no longer tolerate chemically ladened products on my body. One of the products I noticed immediately was self-tanners. Certain brands contained harsh chemicals that dried out my skin and felt toxic to my liver.

So I went on my own journey to seek out healthy self-tanning products that gave me the beautiful golden color I desired and were nourishing to my skin. I was looking for something that could improve the texture and health of my skin as well as enhance the color.

For those of us who are not blessed with naturally rich mocha, chocolate or café au lait skin color, I list a couple of all-natural products that won't poison your body while giving you a beautiful summer glow in the reference section of my book located on my website www.DrElizabeth.com.

Now that you've thoroughly detoxed, it's time to grab your key and step through the next portal gateway, FOOD.

Food

CHAPTER 3

Food

My philosophy on eating and nutrition is simple, put living foods into a living body as often as possible for optimal health, vitality, increased energy and youthfulness.

Decoding the Mystery

There is a vast amount of confusion and misconception around the terms living foods, raw, vegan and vegetarian.

Here's a list of definitions for clarification:

- S.A.D diet- the standard American diet. This includes junk food, fast food, processed food, chemically ladened food, meat, dairy and/or genetically modified food (GMOs).
- Semi-vegetarian- eats no meat except for fish and chicken
- Pesci-vegetarian- eats no meat except for fish
- Lacto-ovo vegetarian- eats no meat, but will eat dairy products (milk, butter, cheese) and eggs
- Ovo-vegetarian- eats eggs, but no meat or dairy products
- Vegan- eats no meat or animal products

THE LINE OF DEMARCATION

- Raw Vegan/ Living Foodist- eats only plant based whole foods and does not heat their food over 118 degrees

Why Living Foods?

Living foods, in their natural state, grown in rich soil, ripened naturally by the sun and picked fresh are bursting with enzymes, minerals, nutrients and amino acids, which are the building blocks of proteins. They are truly perfect foods, which naturally enliven, heal and provide the maximum nourishment possible for the human body.

However, once these foods are cooked above 118 degrees, most of their vital nutrients are denatured and destroyed. I refer to cooked food as "dead food" because of its lack of nutritional value and because it causes the cells in our body to age prematurely.

For these reasons, I feel the best diet possible for maximum health, vitality, radiance and youthfulness is a living foods (raw food) diet. Some people use the term raw food instead of living foods. Both are interchangeable.

The Line of Demarcation Between Health and Disease

Many people believe that the line of demarcation between health and disease lies between a standard American diet (SAD diet) and a vegetarian/vegan diet. And, although that's a great start, I believe that the true line of demarcation between health and disease lies between living foods and cooked (dead) foods.

One of the reasons for the rise in obesity and other food related diseases, such as diabetes, stroke and heart issues, is the consumption of dead (cooked) processed food. Because this food is virtually devoid of nutritional value, even after eating a large meal, the body still wants more. There are several reasons for this physical response.

Dead processed food is ladened with chemicals, excess sodium, sugar and preservatives making it highly addictive. In addition, because this food doesn't nourish the body, it sends a message to the brain saying, "I'm still hungry." This causes an individual to eat more addictive, dead (cooked) processed food and the vicious cycle of weight gain and malnourishment continues resulting in obesity, disease and premature aging.

When people begin to incorporate more living foods into their diet, they naturally release excess weight. The reasons for this phenomenon are two fold. Firstly, the body needs and wants less because it is consuming nutrient dense food. Secondly, they have more energy. This ignites the desire to move their body more often, thus burning more calories.

In addition, today there is an added threat to our food supply with the existence of GMOs (genetically modified organisms). GMO is genetically altered, artificial, un-natural "food" that causes wide spread health challenges. For more information on the dangers that GMOs pose, I recommend watching the documentary film, "Genetic Roulette" created by Jeffrey M. Smith. There are also numerous articles on this subject on the Internet.

It's So Much More Fulfilling and Delicious than a Carrot and a Celery Stick

When I tell people that I consume living foods, most of them imagine that I munch on fruits, veggies, seeds and nuts all day. One of the biggest fears I find with people contemplating a raw/living foods diet is that I'm going to hand them a carrot stick and an apple and say, "Have a nice meal." Truth be told, the scope of living foods is far more expansive, creative and delicious.

As with cooked food, whole living foods can be used to create scrumptious and nutritious meals. The only difference is that the temperature used to prepare these meals is less than 118 degrees to preserve their natural enzymes and nutrients.

Think about it for a minute. If a Jacuzzi is set at 108 degrees, it's virtually too hot to use. That means a meal that has been heated to 118 degrees is HOT.

If you're concerned that you're going to miss out on all your favorite foods, relax. There are an endless number incredible recipes on YouTube and in raw food cookbooks that show you how to prepare "live" versions of your favorite dishes. Trust me, these meals are even more delicious than their cooked versions.

If you live in a large city, there are delightful living/raw food restaurants that offer delicious meals that mimic just about all your favorite standard International and American fare.

In the reference section of my book located on my website, DrElizabeth. com, I provide a list of resources including my favorite youtube videos, books and raw food restaurants located in various cities around the world.

Getting High on Raw Food

The first time I ate prepared living foods I felt tremendously energized. Many people say the same thing. I took a client of mine to one of the local living food restaurants in Los Angeles. She was shocked not only to discover how delicious the food is but that the meal actually made her feel high. She was so astonished by this experience that she went back to the restaurant a couple of days later just to make sure it wasn't a fluke. Sure enough, it wasn't.

The reason that raw/living foods make people feel high is because they are packed with nourishment. People consuming a SAD diet are severely lacking in vital nutrients because these nutriments have been "cooked" out of them.

Living/raw food is so nutrient dense, your body needs very little to be incredibly nourished and energized. The first time your body gets a taste of this kind of food, it's like mainlining pure light energy into your system. I've seen people become giddy and joyous on raw/living foods. But don't take my word… try it yourself.

The Beautiful Italian Gourmet (Not Raw) Food Chef

Meet Lucille, an incredibly beautiful and talented Italian gourmet chef who also just happens to be my Mother. I was inspired to share her story with you because, like many people, Lucille had absolutely no interest or intention in embracing a living foods lifestyle.

My mother is one of those fortunate few who is naturally gifted with beautiful skin and a genetically slender body. When I discovered living foods many years ago, I tried to introduce this way of eating to my mom, but she was not having it. "That's great for you, Elizabeth, but I like my food cooked," she would reply with a gracious, if somewhat patronizing smile.

One day, instead of trying to get her to do the green thing, I decided I would just introduce her to my rich and delicious chocolate milkshake. I didn't even mention that it was "raw." I just brought it over for her to taste and the next thing I knew she was putting in her order for one of my scrumptious shakes on a daily basis.

When I mentioned that this delectable treat was "raw" it piqued her interest. But, it was the powerful cleansing effect of smoothies and juices that really got her to give living foods a try.

Mom is now the proud owner of her very own juicer, which she uses daily. In fact, she recently told me that if she happens to miss a day, she really feels the difference. She confessed that the green juices and smoothies give her much greater energy, more regularity, glowing skin and sparkling eyes. Incorporating these drinks into her diet also caused her to want to eat healthier.

Much to her chagrin, a big bowl of cooked pasta or lasagna that used to put a huge smile on her face, just doesn't sit that well in her tummy anymore. She admits feeling sluggish and groggy the morning following a heavy, cooked meal. Thanks to the incredibly delicious raw food restaurants, she now can feast on yummy Italian dishes, "living foods style," without the negative side effects their cooked versions can cause.

You don't need to eat 100% living foods to get the fabulous benefits that nutrient rich living foods provides. Just by incorporating more of them into your daily diet, you'll look and feel exponentially younger, healthier and certainly more radiant.

Living Foods Lifestyle

What is a living foods lifestyle? I use this term to describe the total enhanced lifestyle that living foods promotes. One of the things I have noticed since embracing living foods and helping others do the same, is that this single shift in eating habits, encourages people to embrace a healthier way of living altogether.

Small Changes = Massive Results

People who consume living foods naturally start exercising more. They become more creative and begin to express more of their innate gifts and talents. Living foods also encourages people to follow their dreams. They become more intuitive and pursue the inner guidance given to them. All the way around, it is an enhanced life experience, which is why I refer to it as a comprehensive living foods lifestyle. Miracles and magic can happen when you embrace this way of living.

"The Substitution Game"

One of the biggest concerns I've noticed with people contemplating a living foods diet/lifestyle is the loss in taste and texture of their food. In response to this matter, I've created "The Substitution Game".

Here's a very simple breakfast substitution as an example of what is possible in the realm of living foods. My hope is that it ignites your creative juices so that you can invent some delicious raw food meals of your own.

Breakfast of Champions

Instead of pouring a bowl of box cereal and cows milk, which are loaded with chemicals, preservatives, hormones and virtually devoid of nutritional value, grab a bowl and fill it with healthy, raw, unprocessed seeds and nuts.

Here's a list of 6 seeds and 6 nuts that are packed with nutrients:

Seeds:

- Chia
- Flax
- Sesame- black or white
- Pumpkin
- Sunflower
- Hemp

Nuts:

- Almonds
- Cashews
- Pecans
- Brazilian nuts
- Hazelnuts
- Walnuts

In the bowl, place whatever combination of seeds and nuts suits your fancy. Add fresh organic fruit such as berries, bananas, mango, etc. Pour homemade almond or any other nut milk over your handmade cereal and enjoy a breakfast that is fit for royalty. This meal will fill your body with energy for the entire morning.

NOTE: Consult your physician or health care provider before making any changes in your diet. Please be aware of any food allergies (including nuts) you may have when embarking on a new diet or eating regimen.

Dr Elizabeth, What do You Eat?

I speak on many raw food panels at various conferences and inevitably someone asks the question, "Dr. Elizabeth, what do you eat?" I love answering this question because I believe if people knew what their healthy food choices were, they would choose wiser and become healthier and happier. Here's a sample of some of my favorites.

Have a Drink

I am a huge proponent of drinking your breakfast. You can pack far more nutrients into a smoothie or raw juice than you can into a bowl or plate of food.

Breakfast

I start out my morning with a living foods juice. It's a fabulous and delicious way of getting your greens for the day. Here's a sample of a typical morning juice:

• Parsley	(1 bunch)
• Spinach	(1 bunch)
• Fuji apple	(1)
• Carrot	(3-4)
• Ginger	(1 inch cube)

(Use organic fruits and vegetables whenever possible)

I simply place each of these items into the juicer and within minutes I have an incredibly energizing juice that fills me with healthy nutrients. You can substitute any other greens such as kale or dandelions instead of parsley or spinach. I also invite you to get creative and make up your own veggie and fruit combinations. It is best to keep the fruit content low and the greens content high for maximum benefits.

"BELIEVE IT OR NOT, GREENS ARE ADDICTIVE."
–Mimi Kirk, Raw Food Exert and Author of "Live Raw Around the World"

One of the things I discovered when I did my juice cleanse and became raw is that greens are addictive. This was a shocking revelation for me. Never in a million years would I have guessed that I would be addicted to healthy nutrient rich greens. I've had an incredible sweet tooth my entire life. In fact, when I was a little girl, I thought heaven consisted of rows and rows of buffet tables overflowing with cookies, cakes, ice cream and candy (not the raw versions) and I was allowed to graze to my heart's content. So no one was more surprised than me to discover that greens are addicting. My body now craves these nutrient rich dynamos on a daily basis.

I invite you to start slow when adding greens to your raw juice. Unless you are dealing with a serious disease, allow your body to get used to the greens. They will grow on you and soon, you too will be craving these in-credible nutrients from Mother Earth and the sea.

Smoothies

I follow the juice with a green smoothie, which I take with me to the gym. Here's a sample of one of my morning smoothies:

- Orange or Pineapple juice base (4 small or 3 large oranges or ½ of a pineapple)
- Frozen banana* (1 large or 2 small bananas)
- Frozen strawberries (6-8 large strawberries)
- Some sort of greens (Kale leaves, parsley, spinach, dandelion)
- Chlorella (Start with ½ to 1 teaspoon)
- Spirulina (Start with ½ to 1 teaspoon
- Green Kamut (Start with ½ to 1 teaspoon)
- Greens Powder of your choice (Start with 1 teaspoon)
- Raw Protein Powder (1 large scoop)

Mix in the blender and within seconds you'll have a delicious and nutritious smoothie.

*Make sure you peel the bananas and cut them into pieces before freezing them. I discovered the hard way that it is incredibly difficult to peel a frozen banana. You only need to cut the bananas if you're using a standard blender. If you have a high-powered blender, this is not necessary.

NOTE: Consult your physician or health care provider before using any potent super foods such as Chorella, Spirulina, Green Kamut and/or Super Greens.

Salads

Salads certainly aren't what they used to be. There are so many incredible greens available in the organic section of the store or farmers market. You can add colorful sweet peppers, tomatoes, sweet peas, ginger, sprouts, seasonal fruit, dried fruit, coconut flakes, herbs, etc. The choices are endless.

What I discovered when I went raw is how delicious and unique each fruit and veggie is when in their wholesome raw form. If you don't believe me, try it yourself. Cut a sweet yellow or orange pepper and take a bite. You'll be amazed at the incredible flavors and textures of these simple and healthy whole foods.

Downloading the Secrets of the Universe in Every Bite

At our core, we are Light. Therefore, the more we nourish our body with light-filled living foods, the more radiant, youthful, beautiful and sexy we become.

Imagine for a second a luscious, ripe bell pepper. This sweet little pepper has been chillin' in the sun soaking up the all the healing light and love energy from the Universe.

Now imagine the roots of this pepper are absorbing all the wisdom and light energy from Mother Earth. So that little pepper is literally filled with the secrets of the Cosmos. Therefore, each time you enjoy a delicious bite, the cells of your body are infused with Universal intelligence, creativity and healing energy.

Next time you reach for an organic fruit or veggie, delight in and give thanks for the beautiful gifts it is giving you.

How are You Going to Dress it Up?

I highly recommend making your own salad dressing. Here's a simple and delicious salad dressing recipe.

- Raw coconut oil or raw extra virgin olive oil (1 tablespoon)
- Apple cider vinegar or any other raw vinegar (2 tablespoons)
- Raspberries or other berries   (1/2 cup of berries)
- Oranges   (The juice from 1 medium orange)
- Fresh veggies   (1 stalk of celery for natural added salt)
- Honey or other raw sweetener   (1 tablespoon)
- Ginger   (I/2 inch square)
- Garlic   (1 clove) optional

Simply place the ingredients in a blender and mix. You can also place in a jar with a lid and shake until mixed.

For more salad dressing or main dish recipes, you can go onto YouTube and place the name of the dish you want to create with the word raw in front of it. For example if you want a lasagna recipe, just place "raw lasagna recipe" in the subject search area and you'll be treated to numerous wonderful recipes from award winning raw food chefs.

Don't Forget the Dessert

One of my favorite raw foods is dessert. There are amazing raw food recipes available to create everything from raw chocolate, cheesecake, chocolate mousse, cookies and more. These dessert treats are absolutely delicious and are a very healthy way to satify a sweets craving.

Super Foods from the Sea

Ocean vegetation provides more minerals than any land veggies. Minerals are vital to our overall health and contribute greatly to our radiance and youthfulness. I make it a point of getting my daily dose of sea veggies for great health and super skin. You can eat them in salads, put them in smoothies or enjoy them as a snack.

Here's a list of a couple of sea vegetables to add to your diet:

- Nori   the seaweed used in sushi rolls
- Dulse   red kelp that you can eat dried
- Wakame   great for making seaweed salads
- Spirulina   blue green algae powder often used in smoothies
- Chlorella   green algae powder often used in smoothies

Check your local Asian Market or the Internet to procure these items and start reaping the rich benefits of nutritious sea veggies today.

Coconut... The Food of the Gods

The coconut is considered by many cultures to be the food of the Gods. This is because each of its components is incredibly nutrient dense. It is also one of my favorite foods.

Coconut Water - Electrolyte Heaven

Coconut water is the liquid inside a young Thai coconut. It is rich in electrolytes and minerals, absolutely delicious and a far better post-workout choice than over the counter sports drinks, which can be loaded with sugars, chemicals and preservatives.

Super Cherry Coconut Juice

For a delicious and refreshing treat try adding dried organic cherries to your coconut water:

- Take 2 cups of coconut water (from a young Thai coconut)
- Add ¾ cup of dried organic cherries*

Let the cherries soak in the water for approximately 15-20 minutes.

*You can substitute other dried fruit instead of dried cherries.

The Magic of Coconut Oil

Raw coconut oil is one of the most perfect oils because it is a medium chain triglyceride (good fatty acids). MCT (medium chain triglycerides) are easily digested and can permeate cell membranes. Coconut oil has been proven to help fight bacteria, viruses, yeast, fungus and candida. In addition, it helps make your skin soft, supple and incredibly touchable.

Coconut Meat for a Great Snack Treat

Coconut meat is rich in vitamins, minerals, antioxidants and fiber. All of these facts make the humble coconut a major beauty bonanza and a one-stop shop for potent nutrition. Try adding coconut meat, coconut water and coconut oil to your next morning smoothie for added energy and a huge beauty boost.

Super Power vs. Regular Power

I am often asked if it is necessary to have a high-powered blender in order to begin a raw food diet. If you're not in a place to make the financial investment in a high-powered blender, a standard blender will suffice. You can save for a fancy blender, but don't let that stop you from reaping the nutritional benefits smoothies and raw foods offer.

Juicer vs. Blender

This is not an either or decision in my opinion. I rate a juicer right up there with a blender as a must have. Again, you can get started with a very inexpensive juicer and save up for a fancier model down the road. Juicing is important because it infuses nutrient dense liquid right into your veins with one sip. I highly recommend this piece of equipment for your kitchen. If you are on a tight budget, I suggest checking garage sales, thrift shops and online websites such as eBay or Craigslist.

Unfortunately, many people become inspired to get healthy and then abandon their undertaking after a couple of months. Because of this fact, you can acquire a wonderful juicer, high-powered blender or dehydrator for a bargain if you take the time and energy to look. Think of it as going on a healthy scavenger hunt.

Dehydrator... the Secret to Creating Really Yummy Raw Food

Dehydrators are used for more than just drying fruit these days. They heat and dry food slowly while keeping the temperature under 118 degrees.

This is a wonderful tool for preparing raw/living food meals. A dehydrator allows you to get really elaborate with your raw food. You can create incredible gourmet entrees, delicious crunchy chips, appetizers and yummy desserts with this piece of equipment.

"EVERY DAY EAT FOODS (AND DRINK BEVERAGES) THAT HAVE BEEN KISSED BY THE SUN AND NOT TAMPERED WITH BY HUMAN HANDS."
–Dr. Michael Beckwith, Spiritual Teacher and Author of "Spiritual Liberation"

Get it Straight From the Source

As often as possible, choose nutrition that has not been processed in any way. For example, instead of purchasing coconut water in a plastic container that has been processed in a plant and hasn't seen the inside of a coconut in weeks, it is far better and more nutritious to buy a young Thai coconut, crack it open and drink the pure fresh coconut water right out of God's cup.

I understand that some of you live in places where this may not always be an option. However, whenever you're able, choose fresh, living, just picked off the tree foods.

Imagine an orange that is basking in the radiant sunlight. It is being fed all the rich nutrients and love from both Mother Earth and Father Sky. You reach up, pick it, bless it and eat it. Your body is immediately filled with pure light energy from the Universe. This is how we were meant to eat. So, whenever possible, grab your nutrition straight from the source. If you can't pick it yourself, local farmers markets are the next best option.

When you choose freshly picked living foods, you exponentially increase the nutritional density of the food you're consuming. Think of it as getting the most "bang for your buck." If you're going to pay good money for good food, you might as well get the most nutrition God put into that food.

Small Shifts Make a Huge Difference

I was talking to my friend, Ron in the gym one day. When I asked him how he was doing, he said that he wished he had more strength and vitality. I tuned into his energy field and noticed that his body was sluggish due to a lack of proper nutrition. Eating heavy foods late at night and consuming an unhealthy breakfast was making him groggy.

I asked if I could make a couple of very simple shifts in the way he was eating and he gratefully consented. I could see that he was eating too much food too close to bedtime so I suggested eating his main meal for lunch and having a light salad for an early dinner. Then I encouraged him not to eat anything else before he went to sleep. In the morning, instead of boxed cereal with milk or oatmeal, which are both "dead" food, I suggested a green fruit smoothie. I invited him to try this for one week and see if he felt better.

The next time I saw him in the gym, he was like a new man. He bragged about having a noticeable increase in vitality. His workouts were a good deal easier thanks to this added boost of energy. He said that he felt much better and more alive. And, his skin even glowed.

If you're feeling a little listless and lethargic, give these simple shifts in your diet a try and let me know if you start having more energy, enthusiasm and vigor.

Give Your Coffee Pot the Day Off

Recently I moved in to a beautiful apartment with a dear friend of mine. When Carol and I moved in together she proudly placed her coffee pot right next to my blender and juicer stating that she'll never give up her morning coffee. I asked her if she'd just be willing to drink a green juice each morning before she made her coffee and see how it made her feel. She agreed.

Much to her surprise, she loved the juice and was amazed how incredible it made her feel. I'm happy to share that the coffee pot has never even been turned on and these days, Carol doesn't want to go a day without her green juice.

There have been many scientific studies showing that giving up coffee assists in weight loss. So if you've been trying to release those last few tenacious pounds or just want to kick start your new healthy living foods lifestyle program, make the swap and watch the scale tip in your favor.

"The Delay Effect"

Ever notice that you'll eat a meal and feel great but then about 20 minutes later you feel "too full?" The reasons for this are receptors in your stomach which register how full you are. Unfortunately, it takes time for these receptors to kick in.

I call this "The Delay Effect" and learning how to counterbalance this digestion factor can assist you in naturally and easily releasing unwanted pounds.

Here are four easy steps to counterbalance "The Delay Effect":

- Slow down- don't eat so fast. Most people are constantly in a rush and don't take time to sit down, eat slowly and enjoy their meal.
- Chew your food- be mindful to consciously and intentionally chew each bite of food sufficiently. This aids in the digestion process.
- Eat smaller servings- Serve your food on a small plate or bowl and reduce your portions.
- Stop eating BEFORE you begin to feel full. This might seem strange the first time you practice this tip, but I promise you, it's one of the best and easiest ways to help you manage your weight. Once you do this a couple of times, your body will get accustomed to, and naturally adopt this technique.

Where Do You Get Your Protein?

This is one of the most commonly asked questions I encounter from people inquiring about a living foods diet/lifestyle. As someone who came from an athletic and fitness background, I wondered the same thing myself. This question kept me from embarking on a living foods lifestyle much earlier than I did. Like many others, I was duped into thinking that my body needed large quantities of animal protein.

The mass media trying to sell you quote-unquote "protein rich foods" wants you to believe this myth. The truth is, what your body really needs are amino acids. Protein is just the middleman. Think about it, what is protein made of...Amino acids. Living foods are a rich source of amino acids. When you eat a diet consisting of living whole foods and super foods, your body gets all the protein it needs.

"WE ARE DESIGNED TO EAT A DIET PRIMARILY MADE UP OF PLANT FOODS: GREENS, FRUITS AND VEGETABLES, SPROUTS, SEEDS AND NUTS. WITH THIS TYPE OF DIET, WE FLOURISH AND DERIVE ALL OUR NECESSARY NUTRIENTS, WHILE ALSO KEEPING OUR BODIES TOXIN FREE AND LOOKING OUR MOST BEAUTIFUL."
–*Kimberly Snyder, Beauty Expert and Author of "The Beauty Detox Solution"*

In Kimberly Snyder's book, "The Beauty Detox Solution," she eloquently explains why we are much closer in our genetic make-up to animals that consume a plant-based diet such as gorillas than we are to animals that are carnivores such as tigers. But, don't worry; you don't need to immediately convert if you've spent your entire life consuming a carnivorous diet.

If you begin to incorporate more living foods into your diet, you will enjoy remarkable benefits. The more you feast on a plant based living foods diet, the more amazing you'll look and feel.

I have worked with numerous clients who swore they'd never give up meat. However, once on a living foods diet, they felt so radiant and healthy, they naturally became vegans without any effort or challenge. Just give it a try… you'll be thrilled you did.

Super Foods for Super Human Capacities

There's been a lot of talk about super foods lately so I'd like to address it here for a minute. Before I do, however, it is important to understand that there are three types of food:

- Food that actually harms you- processed, chemically ladened food,

GMOs, junk food, fast food, etc.
- Food that nourishes/feeds you- fruits, veggies, seeds, nuts
- Food that actually heals you- super foods

"LET FOOD BE THY MEDICINE."
–*Hippocrates, Ancient Greek Physician*

Super Foods fall in the category of foods that actually heal you. If you draw a horizontal line, to the far left end is junk food, processed food and chemically ladened food. On the far right end you'll find super foods and living foods.

The food on the far right side stimulates cell regeneration and enhances life. The food on the far left side causes premature aging and disease. All the whole foods I have been speaking about in this chapter fall under the catagory of nutriments that nourish and heal you.

It's time for people to utilize food for what it has always been intended, a tool to heal, rejuvenate and give life. Begin today by adding more whole living foods to your diet and see for yourself how a living foods lifestyle can help you look and feel years younger.

My Journey to Living Foods

As an athlete, I've been searching for foods that would give me the greatest source of energy and peak performance my entire life.

I come from an Italian background. When I was a little girl, we would gather often at my Grand Mama's home for huge family dinners. My Grandmother would prepare incredible seven course meals. To give you an idea of the breadth and scope of the food served, Lasagna was merely the appetizer.

I remember one particular Sunday, sitting at the table, thinking to myself, "Why are we stuffing ourselves with all of this food only to feel overly full and lethargic afterwards?" I didn't make any sense to me. As much as I enjoyed this delicious food, at eight years old, somehow, I knew that it didn't fuel my body, mind or spirit.

I believe that I came into this lifetime with an inherent interest in healthy eating. This particular experience activated that recollection for me at a very early age.

Over the next several years, I started eating more mindfully. I went on an exploration to discover what foods serve me, or, as my dear friend, raw food chef, Koya Webb says, "Which foods love me back." I eliminated all foods that made me tired and sluggish. I also ate smaller portions, being mindful to stop before I became full. While I was still a pre-teen, I stopped eating French fries, hamburgers, hot dogs, etc. and began eating more fruits and veggies.

Since I was a competitive athlete, I would test the efficacy of the food during my practices. I was a swimmer and springboard diver at the time. I noticed that the healthier the food, the stronger I became. This excited me. I felt I discovered a secret for achieving greater human potentiality.

By the time I was a teenager, I had completely eliminated all junk food. I remember going to lunch with my high school girlfriends. Lunch, for them, consisted of a visit to various local fast food restaurants. I would pull out my fruits and veggies and they would tease me. They're definitely not laughing at me now.

When I went to college, I was one of the few girls who didn't succumb to the "freshman spread." I continued my food experimentation in the University cafeteria. I was already eating salads. My next step was to seek out healthier dressings. I realized that "a salad" loaded with rich fatty dressings defeated the purpose of eating a salad. I replaced the standard iceberg lettuce with greener, leafier more nutritious choices such as spinach, kale, and even dandelion greens.

For many years I ate a diet solely consisting of fish, chicken, fruits and veggies. I was interested in embracing a vegan diet because I care about the wellbeing of my animal brothers and sisters, but as an athlete and avid workout enthusiast, I couldn't figure out how in the world to get my protein.

One day I was invited to do a cleanse with my dear friend, Reirani. At the same time I was working out at the gym with my close friend and teacher, Michael Beckwith. He kept telling me to embrace a vegan diet but I couldn't wrap my brain around eliminating fish and chicken from my diet. I had been a victim of mass media brainwashing. I bought into the myth that my body needed animal protein to be a high performance athlete. As a woman who trains intensely at the gym 2-3 hours a day/ six days a week, and dances several hours a day, I was deeply concerned that I would lose my strength and stamina if I gave up animal protein.

After I finished that cleanse, I couldn't go back to my old diet of chicken and fish. My body and spirit wouldn't allow it.

At the same time, a very dear friend and client, Norman Cohen introduced me to raw food. At almost 77 years young, Norman is the living embodiment of all that is vital, vibrant and youthful. He runs every day, plays basketball at the beach with men half his age and has more energy than most people combined. I am incredibly grateful to Norman for the wealth of knowledge he continues to generously share with me.

In addition to what Norman taught me, I began researching raw food on the Internet. I discovered a great deal of information on YouTube. I was amazed at the number of people who were embracing a living foods lifestyle and the incredible health benefits they were reaping because of that choice.

The turning point for me was when I discovered professional athletes who improved their physical performance, strength and agility after giving up an animal based diet and embracing a raw food diet. One person, whose story really impressed me, is Tim Van Orden.

Tim had been a casual runner his entire life but by the time he was in his late thirties, injuries kept him from his running hobby. After embarking on a raw food diet, he reversed his injuries and began competing in intense marathons and building climbs professionally.

Other individuals who inspired me to make the shift to a raw vegan diet are high endurance professional plant based athletes, Brendan Brazier and Rich Roll. Between the glowing skin, luminous eyes and increased physical performance of raw foodists, such as Tim, Rich and Brendan, that's all I needed to convince me to give this living foods lifestyle a try.

The Benefits of Living Foods

For me, one of the most tangible benefits of a raw food diet was reflected in the glowing faces and remarkable physiques of the raw foodists I met. The advantages of living foods were undeniable. It was written all over their bodies, faces and being.

I decided that raw food was definitely worth the endeavor. I fervently pursued a living foods lifestyle and never looked back.

Get Your Glow On

One of the many benefits I've noticed is the quality of skin tone and texture of people who are on a predominantly plant based/vegan raw food diet. It's undeniable, the beauty benefits of embracing a living foods lifestyle. To me it's worth pursuing for this fact alone.

Increased Clarity, Clairvoyance, Creativity and Intuition

But that's just the beginning. What I also noticed is tremendous clarity, intuition, wisdom, clairvoyance and expanded creativity. People I met who consumed living foods not only glowed on the exterior; they were luminous from the inside out. They seemed to be more joyous, peaceful, alive and enthusiastic. They also took great care and concern for humanity and Mother Earth. They had careers that were in tremendous service to others and the planet and were very loving and compassionate human beings.

Here are some fabulous benefits to a living foods lifestyle:

- Incredible Energy
- Proper Weight Stabilization
- Tremendous Mental Clarity
- Increased Intuition
- Greater Capacity to Love and Be Loved
- Balanced Emotions
- Elimination of Disease
- Desire to Discover and Live Your Purpose
- Desire to Make a Difference in the World

Some people, when they discover living foods, dive in. It can be quite an ordeal as your body goes through its detoxification process. However, most people move slowly from a SAD (standard American diet) to living foods. I invite you to move at your own pace and allow your body and your spirit to lead the way.

When you adapt these concepts and practices into your daily life, this new fountain of youth lifestyle will give you more enthusiasm, energy, vitality, vibrancy and fun than you ever thought possible.

Now that you have the key to access youth promoting nutrition, let's step through the next portal to the fountain of youth... MOVEMENT.

Move

CHAPTER 4

Move

66"WHEN WE MOVE OUR BODIES IN WAYS THAT GIVE US GREAT JOY, FROM WORK-ING OUT TO MAKING LOVE, WE MARRY OUR SPIRIT WITH OUR PHYSICAL BODY FOR A HUMAN EXPERIENCE THAT IS DIVINE."
–Dr. Elizabeth Lambaer, Inspirational Speaker and Author of "Skinny Dipping in the Fountain of Youth"

Longevity vs. Youthfulness

There's a great deal of talk these days about longevity. While I feel that it is important to live a long life, to me, what good is longevity if it is not accompanied by vitality and youthfulness? Therefore, I prefer to use the word youthfulness instead of longevity.

Flexibility- the Key to Youthfulness

Have you ever noticed how much energy is released every time you stretch?

Flexibility is one of the biggest keys to youthfulness. When a traumatic experience occurs, the energy of that experience is stored in the body. If it is not cleared, it can cause numerous challenges, physically, mentally, emotionally and spiritually. When you stretch your muscles, you release old energy lurking in the memory banks of your cells, leaving you feeling calm, peaceful and clear. Think of it as meditation for the body.

Flexibility in the body reflects flexibility in the mind, heart and spirit. Yoga and Pilates are wonderful stretching practices. Check out the classes being offered at your local gym or studio, stretch on your own or with a partner. Make it one of your daily healthy habits and watch your stress levels diminish and your flexibility expand.

When I turned 50, one of my personal goals was to exponentially increase my flexibility. Mass consciousness tells us that our flexibility dwindles as we circle the sun each year. My intention was to prove mass consciousness wrong. And that is exactly what I did.

At 55 years young, I am more flexible than ever. People often ask me, "How can I improve my flexibility?" I'm delighted to share my secret stretching exercise in order to help you increase your flexibility.

Flexibility Enhancement Exercise

This exercise will help you improve your 2nd splits (Chinese splits) flexibility. If you are interested in enhancing your flexibility in other areas of your body, apply the techniques used in this exercise. Simply position your body according to the specific area you wish to stretch.

Lay down on a mat or soft surface such as a carpet or mattress. Place your buttock against a wall and extend your legs out in a Y position. (See photo on next page)

For an added stretch, lay on a foam roller while doing this exercise. That will place you in a position to stretch your neck, back and shoulders as well. Take caution when positioning yourself so you don't roll off the foam roller.

Close your eyes and begin taking long, slow, deep yoga breaths. Place your right hand on your stomach and your left hand on your heart. Follow your breath as instructed in the meditation exercise outlined in chapter 2, HEAL (page 44).

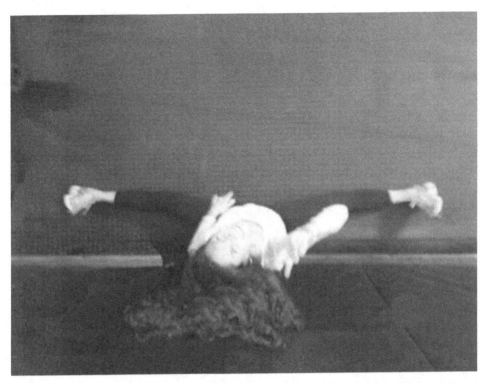

Demonstration of the Proper Position for Chinese/2nd Splits Stretching Exercise (While Laying on a Foam Roller)

Now place all of your attention and energy in your 6th chakra (in the center of your head). Light it up with a beautiful bright starburst of light energy like an explosion of fireworks in the night sky.

With your energy and focus still on your 6th chakra, look down (from within your body) to your 1st chakra (at the base of your spine) and light it up like a starburst of light energy. Create a grounding cord from the bottom of your 1st chakra all the way down to the center of the earth. Your grounding cord is what connects you to Mother Earth. You can use any image you'd like to create your grounding cord. Some examples include, a strong oak tree, a beam of light, a string of pearls, a steel beam or a waterfall. Use your imagination to find a grounding cord image that works best for you.

Once your grounding cord is down and you feel connected and grounded to the earth, place your focus on the area where your legs connect to your hip sockets. Draw an imaginary energetic triangle between your hipbones and the base of your spine.

For women, this area contains your female genitalia and for men, your male genitalia. This area can hold a lot of energetic wounding around intimate relationships and/or sexual experiences especially for women. When a woman experiences hurt or pain in some form resulting from these experiences, those memories can be stored in her physical body causing limited flexibility. The same can hold true for men.

Think of every past lover, boyfriend, girlfriend, husband, wife or any other person you have been intimate with who has hurt you. Pick one individual at a time and send that pain and all the memories associated with those painful experiences down the grounding cord and give it to the earth. See Mother Earth receiving all of that pain in her loving arms and transforming it into the energy of love. From the vantage point of your 6th chakra, take your time and really see the energy flowing from that triangle between your hipbones and sit bone all the way down the grounding cord.

You can also place an imaginary movie screen at eye level, about 2 feet in front of you. Sometimes it is easier to view this clearing process from the perspective of this movie screen.

With your focus and attention still in your 6th chakra, look down and see your 4th chakra, your heart chakra, (in the center of your chest). Light it up like a star burst. Now imagine waves of loving energy flowing up from Mother Earth and filling your entire being with healing energy.

Do the same thing with your 7th chakra (at the top of your head) and invite healing Cosmic energy from Father Universe to flow into you from the top of your head. Feel and see these energies merging and swirling together in a sparkling radiant light and filling your body with tremendous love. Allow that love to fill each one of your chakras starting at the top of your head (7th chakra) and moving all the way down to the base of your spine (1st chakra).

Now imagine a golden sun above your head. Fill this sun with your own beautiful energy. Then invite in the energy of love, light and whatever you wish to bring into your being and physical body right now. If you wish to call forth a loving intimate relationship or any other manifestation that is in your heart, place these desires into this golden sun. Once you fill up your golden sun, reach up above your head and begin to bring this radiant ball of light and love into your body. Imagine pure luminescent golden liquid pouring into the top of your head. See it flowing into your entire body. Feel it and welcome it into every cell of your being and let it completely wash over you and continue all the way down your grounding cord into Mother Earth. Take a minute to bask in this blissful light. Do this for each relationship where you experienced hurt, pain and heartache.

Ask your body if it is holding any other painful energy and memories associated with those experiences. Invite your body to let go of whatever it is ready to release. You don't even need to remember what the painful memory was, once your body is ready to release it, it will naturally and automatically do so during this exercise.

As you do this, feel the opening in the triangle between your hipbones and sit bone. Do this every time you stretch and watch your flexibility increase exponentially. You can do this exercise for every part of the body you desire to increase flexibility.

The key to the success of this exercise remains in remembering that emotional wounding and memories are stored in the physical body causing it to tense up, become rigid and stiff, aging you prematurely. A physical body that is free of those traumatic memories is supple, flexible and youthful. When you release the mental and emotional energy, the body regains its youthful agility. The release of those old painful memories will also be reflected in your enhanced beauty and radiance.

NOTE: This exercise was inspired by my teacher, Vicki Reiner's grounding exercise.

Move Your Body for the Sheer Joy of it

Movement is absolutely vital to your health and wellbeing. Most adults, many teens and children do not get nearly enough exercise on a daily basis.

The simplest way to correct this situation is to find the types of movements that give you the most joy and then make the commitment to incorporate these specific types of exercise into your daily routine. You'd never dream of leaving your home in the morning without brushing your teeth. It's a healthy habit that is ingrained into your daily lifestyle. It is the same thing with exercise. Once you make exercise a healthy habit, you wouldn't dream of skipping it. Nor should you once you read this startling fact...

"THE FAILURE TO EXERCISE 3 TIMES A WEEK IS THE EQUIVALENT OF SMOKING A PACK OF CIGARETTES A DAY."
–U.S. Surgeon General

I hear people all the time tell me that they don't have time to exercise. The truth is, you don't have time not to exercise. The price that it costs you in sick days, lethargy, depression, weight gain, financial costs, premature aging, loss of sexual prowess and a host of other challenges far outweighs the 30 minutes 3 times a week it takes to just get your body moving.

And if you can't find 30 minutes 3 times a week, start with 15-20 minutes 2 times a week. Like most things in life, I find the secret to success is just to take the first step. Once you feel those delicious endorphins flooding your body, you'll find a way to make that experience a part of your daily life more and more often.

I invite you to pull out your calendar and make a date with yourself or better yet, a friend, to begin or reignite your healthy workout habit today.

Maybe you don't exercise because you haven't found a workout that you're really passionate about. If that's the case...

Go On an Adventure to Discover What Kind of Movements Turn You On

Ask yourself what you loved to do physically when you were a little boy or girl? Did you horseback ride, swim, dance, run, bicycle, skateboard, ski or snowboard?

If you loved it then, you'll love it now. When you love doing something, you naturally want to get up and go do it. And, you'll do it more often and for longer periods of time because it gives you such joy.

Now I can hear some of you saying, there's no way I can get out there and horseback ride, swim or dance again. I'm too "old" and "out of shape" for that sort of thing. As you start detoxing and properly nourishing your body, it will naturally level off at its perfect size and shape and you'll be shocked at what your physical body will be able to do for you again. And if you're thinking that you possess too many nagging aches and pains to exercise, you'll be surprised to discover that a living foods lifestyle along with proper physical, mental and emotional detoxification can heal and reverse many of those ailments.

Remember the story in the previous chapter about Tim Van Orden? He went from a retired runner, due to old nagging leg injuries before he became raw, to a champion runner and tower runner (athletes who run up the stair wells of sky scrapers) since becoming raw vegan. Tim will be the first to tell you, if he can do it, so can you.

And, professional plant based vegan ultra athlete, Rich Roll's story is equally inspiring. On the eve of his 40th birthday, he was 50 lbs overweight and unable to climb a single flight of stairs without becoming winded. After shifting to a plant based vegan lifestyle, he went on to become one of the world's top 25 fittest men and ultra marathon champion.

"LOVE IS THE GREATEST HEALING POWER I KNOW. LOVE CAN HEAL EVEN THE DEEP-
EST AND MOST PAINFUL MEMORIES BECAUSE LOVE BRINGS THE LIGHT OF UNDER-
STANDING TO THE DARKEST CORNERS OF OUR HEARTS AND MINDS."
–*Louise L. Hay, Entrepreneur and Author of "You Can Heal Your Life"*

I have discovered that every physical ailment has an emotional and mental component. When the emotional and mental issues are addressed, the
physical challenge often dissipates. I've seen this time and time again with
my clients.

Louise Hay wrote a wonderful book called, "You Can Heal Your Life"
in which she outlines the emotional components to common physical ailments. I encourage you to use her book as a reference to help you heal whatever physical challenges may be standing in the way of you fully enjoying,
expressing and exercising your beautiful body.

By simply applying the principles I outline in this book, you can enjoy
the thrill and joy of passionate exercise your entire life. It is much easier
than you think to regain your youthful vitality, strength and stamina. Begin
by shifting the way you think from, that's impossible, to that's completely
possible, and you'll be amazed at what your body will do for you.

I invite you to go on an adventure to discover what physical expressions
light you up and give you tremendous joy. Once you find those things, treasure them, woo them like a lover and practice them as often as possible.
Like compound interest, your physical activities will love you back in exponential dividends.

Now I can hear some of you saying, "That's great Dr. Elizabeth, but I
have kids, a high pressure, time consuming career, a husband or wife (or
maybe you're a single mom or dad). How in the world am I going to find
the time to do something for me?"

Well, if you love your children, your family and yourself, you'll find the
time. Do it for your loved ones, if you can't yet find a way to do it for yourself.

Actions speak louder than words. Children mimic what we do, not what we say. When a child, spouse or loved one sees you taking loving actions to care for your physical, mental, emotional and spiritual well being, they learn to do the same thing for themselves. And isn't that what you want for them?

When you begin to take the time to relish in your passionate physical expression, you'll be much happier and your family will be much better off for you having done this, trust me.

Get off the Sideline and Get in the Game

When you take your kids to the park to play, instead of sitting on the park bench, smart phone in hand, texting or talking, put on your play clothes and go out and play with your kids. You can't imagine what 20 minutes on the playground will do, not only for your body but for your mind, heart and spirit as well.

Those 20 minutes will not only refresh and invigorate, they'll provide a fabulous source of exercise. You'll experience a euphoric high from all the endorphins you'll naturally release. In addition, it's a wonderful way to bond with your children. Remember how special it was when you were little and your parents came out and played with you? Your kids are going to love you for it.

A very dear friend of mine, Gail Larkin is a brilliant entrepreneur. She is also a wife and mother to a beautiful 4-year-old daughter. Gail credits her fabulous post-baby body to spending time at the park running around playing with her daughter, Imani. She swears that just their playtime together has done wonders for her physical strength, stamina and the return of her pre-baby physique. And it can do the same for you.

Swing on the Swings

When was the last time you swung on the swings? Do you remember how much fun it was? When was the last time you did that with your kids? Now I don't mean watch them or push them on the swings. I mean when was the last time you actually got on the swings and soared to your hearts content?

As a single woman, I always take a man I'm interested in dating to the playground. I know that might sound silly, but the way he reacts says a lot about his capacity for fun, joy and spontaneity. A person's capacity to express these qualities is directly related to their proclivity towards youthfulness. These qualities are very important for my mate to possess because I'm interested in someone who will match my level of play, joy and fun in our relationship.

If you're single, I invite you to bring your dates to the park for some playtime. It's a great way to stay young and beautiful. It is also incredibly sexy. And, it's surprisingly fabulous foreplay.

One of the things I love best about swinging on the swings is the level of noncausal joy, love and fun I experience. What I mean by noncausal is that these feelings don't come from getting something from the outside world.

For example, when I swing on the swings, I am not happy because of a new job, a new boyfriend or winning the lottery. I am simply filled with joy, love and fun just because I am delighting in the experience of being alive.

Some of you have experienced noncausal joy and love watching a beautiful sunset or at the birth of your child. These divine qualities are our innate state of being. They come standard with every body. There are so many things in life that don't cost a penny that can help you experience joy, love and fun. Swinging on the swings is just one of them.

In my work with private clients, one of the things I notice is that they all speak about this insidious itch that can't be scratched. They are very successful, prominent, beautiful women and men who, from the outside world, appear to have it all. And yet, behind closed doors, they confess to me that they are secretly longing for more joy, love and fun in their life.

"The JLF Factor"

The juiciness you experience from the divine qualities of Joy, Love and Fun is what I lovingly refer to as, "The JLF Factor." This secret X factor is one of the greatest and quickest pathways to the fountain of youth.

I began to cultivate this idea of the Joy Factor, the Love Factor and the Fun Factor because I was having incredible success using these techniques with my clients. I witnessed first hand the radical difference applying these factors had on their lives. I see them as tools that, when applied to any life, bring immediate, exponential and permanent increases in radiance, passion, youthfulness, vitality, sex appeal, abundance and wellbeing.

There are numerous other benefits of embracing "The JLF Factor." The energies of joy, love and fun vibrate at such a high frequency that when you immerse yourself in this field of energy, you automatically magnetize to you everything you've ever wanted, hoped for and dreamed of.

So how can you incorporate "The JLF Factor" into your life?

Exercise #7 "The JLF Factor" Exercise

Carve out an hour in your schedule. If you can make more time, that's great, if you can only spare 20 minutes to ½ hour, that's fine as well.

Take yourself on a play date. You can do this solo or you can invite your kids, your entire family, your friends or anyone who is willing to come along and play with you.

Pick something that is outside the box of what you'd normally do for fun. For example, if you already go to an African dance class, that doesn't count as a play date. On the other hand, if you secretly long to take a Brazilian samba dance class and you've never stepped foot in a dance studio, that would definitely qualify as a wonderful play date.

Challenge yourself to choose something outside your comfort zone. Get creative. Think of things that you've always wanted to do because it sounds so fun but never made the time to do them. Here are some examples of play dates.

"The JLF Factor" play date ideas:

- Fly a kite
- Go to the beach and swim or boogie board (I did this one recently and had the time of my life)
- Go sailing
- Roller skate (make sure to remember your elbow, wrist and knee pads)
- Ride a bike
- Swing on the swings
- Go for a walk in a garden and take time to smell the roses (I mean this literally)
- Watch a really funny movie
- Go to the zoo, an aquarium or a museum
- Draw funny pictures
- Bungee Jumping
- Play I-Spy
- Study Quantum Physics

The only other requirement of this exercise is that it is fun for you. Don't allow someone else to dictate your definition of fun. If it makes you happy, then go for it. Observe how you feel during your adventure. Notice the heightened levels of joy, love and fun you are naturally experiencing. This is how you are meant to feel all the time, every day of your life.

Let me repeat that again, "This is how you are meant to feel all the time, every day of your life!"

"No problem can be solved from the same level of consciousness that created it."
–Albert Einstein, Physicist, Philosopher and Nobel Prize Winner

During your play date, observe how any challenges that might have been on your mind, simply dissipate. This is because you cannot experience fear while in the energy of joy, love and fun. Those divine qualities lift you out of the low vibrational field of fear and place you perfectly in your natural state of being, which is bliss.

As Albert Einstein so eloquently stated in the above quote, getting into an elevated state of being is actually the perfect way to "solve" any challenge that you might be experiencing. From that elevated vibrational frequency, answers that you couldn't have possibly seen, heard or uncovered in your lower vibration frequency synchronistically reveal themselves to you, sometimes in very amusing and refreshing ways.

Afterwards, write in a journal how you felt during your play date in as much detail as possible. Pull out your calendar and schedule another fun adventure within a week. Soon you'll be wondering how you ever got along without "The JLF Factor" (joy, love and fun) in your life.

Change it Up

Part of the fun of exercising is the excitement of a new challenge. Whether you are pushing yourself to the next level or cultivating a new sport, it is important to keep yourself on the edge of expansion when it comes to physical exercise.

Gratitude

I hear people all the time say, "Oh, I have to go to the gym," like it were some sort of burden. I say to them, "No, not so." It is a privilege to be in these human bodies and to be able to move and experience the sheer joy of being alive. I invite you to take a moment and just be thankful for your physical body. Here's a wonderful exercise that will help remind you of the miracle that you are and get you moving when you may not feel up to exercising.

Exercise #8 The Gratitude Exercise

Sit or lay down in a comfortable position. Close your eyes and take a couple of long, slow, deep yoga breaths. Place your attention in your 6th chakra (in the center of your head). With your attention still in your 6th chakra, look down at your 1st chakra (at the base of your spine) and attach your grounding cord from the base of your 1st chakra firmly down into Mother Earth. Bring the energy from Mother Earth up through your feet chakra and into your body. Now look up to your 7th chakra (the top of your head) and invite the energy from Father Universe into your body. Merge the energies from the earth and the universe together in your 4th chakra, your heart chakra. (In the center of your chest)

With great love and appreciation, bring into your mind's eye your kidneys. Bless them and thank them for the amazing job they do filtering fluids in your body every day. Now move on to your heart. Thank it for continuously pumping blood through your body, keeping you alive. Do this with each one of your precious organs. Then move onto your senses, i.e. eyes, ears, nose, throat, skin and thank each one for bringing in the messages from the world. Don't forget your 6th sense.

As you do this, a powerful sense of gratitude for this extraordinary machine called your physical body will begin to well up in you. Really stay in the awe and magnificence of this miracle called you. This is the only body you will receive this lifetime. Do your best to take care of, love and cherish it.

Many people take better care of their possessions than they do their bodies. The next time you don't feel like exercising or eating healthy, remember how incredible your body is and be in gratitude of all that it does for you. Doesn't it deserve to be taken care of to the best of your ability?

To Gym or Not to Gym… that is the Question

You don't have to go to the gym. There are plenty of wonderful and creative ways to get your exercise beyond the four walls of a gym.

Now, I happen to adore going to the gym. I love working out and I love my gym. I go at the same time every morning and visit with my wonderful friends. For me, it's much more than just a time to exercise. I have been going to this gym for almost twenty years. We are a community and these people are my family. I also have amazing training partners. Our workout time together is fun and productive.

"The Updraft Factor"

One of the many benefits of going to the gym is what I call "The Updraft Factor." This effect is based on the dynamic of drafting. Just like birds that fly in formation or cyclists who ride together, human beings can utilize "The Updraft Factor" to take them further than they could possibly go on their own.

People come from all over the world to work out at Gold's Gym in Venice, California. The individuals who workout there are committed to expanding their fitness level and from the moment you walk in the gym this elevated energy is palpable and contagious.

Harnessing and contributing to the collective energy is what "The Updraft Factor" is all about. Every time I exercise, I tap into this energy field and it always helps me workout harder and stronger than I could on my own accord.

There are days when I'm bursting with energy, and I know that my presence contributes to the workouts of those around me. Then there are other days when I could use a little boost of energy, so I utilize the energy that is flowing through the gym in abundance to source and fuel my workout.

"The Updraft Factor" is one of the tools I teach to help people manifest much more in much less time with grace, ease and fun. This technique isn't limited to exercising. You can use it in every area of your life where you'd like to manifest with greater efficiency.

This practice works when you come together intentionally with others and agree to share your energy. Examples are workout partners, business partners, study groups, etc. The other way you can tap into "The Updraft Factor" is by harnessing the available energy in any environment, such as my gym example above. Once you become clear in your own energy field as outlined in chapter 2, HEAL, honing into the energy in any environment becomes simple. Here are some examples of the many environments you can harness; airports, stores and nature. The possibilities are endless.

It is important to remain mindful of the shared flow of energy when utilizing this technique. You don't want to become an energy vampire. Always be mindful to give as well as receive energy when it is shared collectively.

I have always loved the idea of collaboration, co-creation, and the spirit of community. In the mathematics of humanity, one plus one always equals infinity. When two or more come together in the spirit of community, co-creation and collaboration, exponentially greater results occur.

If the thought of exercising, or anything else for that matter seems daunting to you, give this technique a try.

Where can you incorporate the practice of "The Updraft Factor" in your own life? Make a list of the areas in your life where you could begin to incorporate this powerful technique.

- _____
- _____
- _____
- _____
- _____

Who can you contact today to join forces using "The Updraft Factor" to accomplish your dreams and wishes?

- _____
- _____
- _____
- _____
- _____

The Testosterone Spa

One of my girlfriends recently asked me, "Why do you love going to the gym so much?" Then she secretly confessed, "I don't really enjoy it." I answered, "Imagine a place where the odds for women are stacked four guys to every girl. The place is packed with gorgeous, sexy men and oozing with testosterone. A woman could get a contact high from all the testosterone in the place. Now imagine that those men are nice, charming, funny, fun to be around and really appreciative of your presence in the gym. Talk about inspiring. Sounds like a pretty good way to spend an hour or so, a couple of times a week, don't you think?"

She replied, "I never thought of it that way before." After our conversation, I brought her to the gym with me and she had a fabulous time.

For me, going to the gym is exciting, sexy and fun. The men in the gym welcome me with open arms and open hearts. I am a woman who enjoys and appreciates swimming in a sea of testosterone. For me, basking in masculine energy is delicious and makes me feel protected, feminine and free.

I shared that story in an interview I conducted with Love, Relationship and Communications Expert, Alison Armstrong. What ensued is a delicious conversation about the benefits of women being able to embrace the testosterone energy and express their Divine Feminine essence around men.

Alison has dedicated over twenty six years to the study of men, women and how they relate to, and communicate with one another. One of the beautiful things she has discovered is that most men want to contribute to and protect women. It is a desire that is literally encoded in their DNA. The challenge is that some women are unaware of this fact. And, because of this, many fear that testosterone is dangerous. This fear causes enormous challenges in their relationships with men.

"How we [men] demonstrate love is what I call the three P's of love: we profess, we protect and we provide."
–*Steve Harvey, Talk Show Host and Author of "Act Like a Lady, Think Like a Man"*

Alison went on to explain in more detail by saying, "The fear of testosterone is due, in part, to the fact that these women do not fully understand the strength of a man's need to protect a woman." She then shared, "Dr. Elizabeth, when you walk into the gym, your perception is that you are surrounded by protectors, and that's very powerful. You're in your feminine expression, you feel protected and completely safe and therefore, you get high on testosterone."

Alison continued, "Another woman who thinks testosterone is dangerous can walk into the same gym. Because she doesn't feel safe, she will unintentionally put her guard up. As a result, she'll become more masculine, more self-conscious of her body and her need to be physically perfect, and she'll push away the very energy (masculine male energy) that she so deeply desires to attract. She'll be in misery in the same environment that fills Dr. Elizabeth, nurtures her and becomes her personal testosterone spa."

How can a woman begin to shift her perception of men so that she can find comfort and nourishment frolicking in the Testosterone Sea?

"It's about causing a shift in perception so that a woman can live in a world surrounded by protectors so she experiences being safe all the time."
–*Alison Armstrong, Relationship Expert and Author of "The Queen's Code"*

Testosterone Spa Rules

Here are a couple of ways women can begin to embrace the testosterone energy. These rules don't just apply to women who are single. It is important and healthy for all women to learn how to embrace masculine energy:

- Start by recognizing that the masculine energy wants to give, or as Steve Harvey puts it in his book, "Act Like a Lady, Think Like a Man," wants to profess (their love for you), protect and provide.
- Begin to build your trust in men by surrounding yourself with men who you know to be safe and practice allowing them to give to you and protect you.
- Once you have a sense of safety around men, relax your masculine energy and allow your softer, more gentle feminine essence to emerge.
- Start going places where there is an abundance of testosterone i.e. the gym, sports clubs, athletic events, etc. Bring a trusted male friend or girlfriend with you for support. Practice being in your feminine energy and relish in the flurry of delicious masculine attention and admiration that ensues.
- At the same time, hone your discernment. There are a few men out there who may not have the most honorable intentions. The more you are in your feminine essence, the greater access you'll have to your intuition. Allow that inner knowing to inform and guide you to the right men.

Femininity, Masculinity and Sexuality

Some of you may be wondering how to step into your feminine energy. Before answering that question, let's define feminine and masculine energy.

'FEMININE SEXINESS IS HOW RADIANT IS YOUR LIFE FORCE... WHAT IS SEXINESS IS THE FULLNESS OF LIFE FORCE FLOWING THROUGH A WOMAN."
–David Deida, Intimacy Expert and Author of "The Way of the Superior Man"

Over 80% of all women express predominantly from their feminine essence and over 80% of all men express predominantly from their masculine essence.

- Masculine essence/energy is active. It is giving, moving, doing.
- Feminine essence/energy is passive. It is receiving, flowing, being.

One of the greatest tools in a woman's treasure chest of youthfulness and sex appeal is her femininity. There is nothing more delicious to the outside world than a woman who is fully in her feminine expression. She is juicy, sexy, radiant, beautiful, youthful, free and wildly appealing to all those who cross her path. In fact, a woman in her feminine essence is absolutely undeniable regardless of her age. I've experienced this many times in my own life and seen it brilliantly demonstrated time and time again with other women.

"MASCULINE SEXINESS IS NOT LIFE FORCE, INSTEAD, THE MASCULINE IS FEARLESS CONSCIOUSNESS, EMPTY CONSCIOUSNESS, IT'S THE CAPACITY TO BE PERFECTLY PRESENT WITHOUT RECOIL... IT IS ULTIMATELY FEARLESS CONSCIOUSNESS AND TOTAL PRESENT-NESS."
–David Deida, Intimacy Expert and Author of "The Way of the Superior Man"

For a man, being in his masculinity is the key to his youthfulness and sex appeal. That expression of masculine energy will look quite different than a woman's expression of her feminine energy. A man is very sexy and appealing when he has the power to stand fully in his awakened consciousness and powerfully hold the space, like a deep and soulful cauldron, for a woman to flow all of her feminine energy.

Masculine energy is like the solid, immovable, well-constructed building that stands strong in midst of a raging hurricane. The masculine is the building and the feminine is the rush of Mother Nature. Women want to know that a man can hold the totality of their being, their passionate emotions, expressions and fluctuations without flailing in the wind or caving in.

Men and women have within them both masculine and feminine essence. However, in our day-to-day busy lives, both men and women express far more from their masculine than from their feminine energy.

Over the past several decades, there has been a significant increase in the number of women in the workplace. There are more women in positions of power than ever before. This advancement is not only important for women, it is also vital for society. The world is in great need of the Divine Feminine essence in governments, corporations and other places of leadership.

Studies show that societies and businesses that have a more balanced number of women and men in leadership positions, and therefore have greater balance between masculine and feminine energy, are thriving much more than those that don't. It is obvious that the inclusion of women in places of power has been a tremendously positive thing. However, most women have paid a very high price for their success.

More females than ever before spend most of their time expressing from the masculine essence as career women, mothers (yes mothering is a masculine quality) and managing a home and family. They can get lost in the riptide of masculine energy overload.

Most people assume that mothering is a feminine quality. This is a huge misconception. The act of mothering is predominantly caretaking, which is the energy of giving to someone else. Most women make the mistake of thinking that giving is a feminine quality however this is not true. Giving is always a masculine expression.

In intimate relationships, women often make the mistake of over-giving. However, since giving is a masculine quality, this action actually emasculates masculine essence men and pushes them away.

It is a very delicate dance being a powerhouse woman in the world and a feminine essence woman in intimate relationship. The woman who discovers the secret to this balance experiences great success and happiness in both worlds.

Even Superwoman Needs a Helping Hand Every Now and Again

When women went to work, somehow they got the memo to put on their Superwoman cape. No one questioned it, so, for the past 40 plus years, most women have been operating from overdrive and overload. They've been giving at work, giving at home, giving to their kids, giving to their friends, giving to their beloved and never slowing down long enough to receive. This idea of having to be superwoman caught on like wildfire and it's been a crazy rat race ever since.

The challenge with all of these wonderful female advancements is that when a feminine essence woman continuously expresses from her masculine, she becomes exhausted, depleted and unappealing. Even the most physically beautiful woman can become worn out and haggard looking if she spends too much time in her masculine energy, if she is a feminine essence woman. She also subconsciously ends up repelling the masculine energy that she so needs and longs to connect with to nourish and heal because she is constantly in her own masculine expression.

I have many successful, business women come to me because they're not happy. Their careers are at an all time high but their love lives, physical bodies and other elements in their life are at an all time low. They're looking for relief but they don't even know what from or where to begin to find it.

It is vitally important and healing for a woman to take time to relish in her feminine essence in order to maintain balance, beauty and sanity. It is also the place where she magnetizes what she wants to create.

How to Get Your Sexy Back

Many women I meet tell me that they long to feel like a woman again. They've lost their femininity and sex appeal and they want to know how to get their sexy back. Whether they just had a baby, they're going through a divorce, they're dissatisfied with their body or their appearance, they're stressed at work or they're having a difficult time in life, whatever the reason, they don't feel their feminine, sexy best.

It is a woman's essential nature to be absolutely undeniable when she is in her authentic feminine energy. It is also tremendously nourishing. What I suggest is to start by appreciating where you are right now. True femininity and sex appeal have nothing to do with appearance or circumstances. When a woman truly comprehends this fact, she becomes absolutely gorgeous.

The next step is to receive. Everything you most deeply desire is available to you when you allow the energy of receiving into your life. This is a huge part of embracing your feminine side.

I invite you to adopt patience as you allow yourself the gift of receiving. It may feel very foreign to you, even selfish at first. That's okay, just breathe and let it in.

Ladies, it's delicious being a woman. Relish in this precious gift. Delight in all the little things that help make you feel more feminine. Embrace these practices wholeheartedly and allow them to assist you in feeling like the Queen you are again. As you step fully into owning your feminine essence, remember to be kind to yourself as you travel on this exciting journey.

Here are some simple yet powerful tools to help you switch from being super woman who is running the world all day long to super feminine woman who is fully capable of relishing in her soft, sexy feminine essence.

Exercise #9 Techniques to Reclaim Your Feminine Essence

- Take a bath
- Take a walk
- Take a breath
- Talk with a friend
- Spend time in nature

- Put on some music and dance in your home
- Put on some sexy lingerie (whatever that means to you)
- Open up to receive, a gift, a massage, a smile, a hug, etc.
- Take a sexy dance class, pole-dancing class, belly dancing class, salsa dancing, anything that gets your hips moving and shaking

The Hips Don't Lie

"OH BABE, I'M ON TONIGHT, MY HIPS DON'T LIE AND I'M STARTING TO FEEL YOU BOY... COME ON LET'S GO, REAL SLOW, BABY, LIKE THIS IS PERFECTO."
–*Shakira, Award Winning Singer/Songwriter, Performer and Entrepreneur*

Another powerful way for women to tap into their feminine essence and get their sexy back is to move their hips. The 2nd chakra, home of your sensuality, sexuality, femininity (masculinity for men) and creativity is housed in between your hipbones in the area just south of the belly button. If that chakra is shut down, you cannot freely express these qualities.

The other curious thing is that when you restrain one of the qualities in your 2nd chakra, or any other place in your body for that matter, they all become suppressed. For example, if you were raised in a family environment that was puritanical, you might have learned to repress your sexuality. That action, whether it was conscious or unconscious, will cause you to curtail your precious creativity, sensuality and femininity (for women) or masculinity (for men) as well. Likewise, when you suppress your anger and rage it also suppresses your capacity for expressing and feeling joy and bliss.

Today there still exists a double-edged sword regarding sexual expression in our society. In its most exaggerated forms, it is prostituted in the media or pushed down by puritanical control. These are both different sides of the same coin. Both extremes are still locked up in the shame and the shadow side of sexuality.

Freedom of sexual expression is true balance. I find that many women coming from the corporate world have had to push down their natural feminine, sensual and sexual expression in the workplace. Many have had to dress like men and try to fit into a man's world. These women are hungry to freely express their femininity. Moving the hips unlocks the energy, allows the feminine essence to flow and is one of the best ways to regain your juicy radiance and youthfulness.

The beauty of reawakening your sexual articulation is that is gives you access to one of the greatest gifts a human being possesses, your creative imagination. If you've felt stifled creatively, look at where you may be suppressing other emotions in your life. If this resonates with you, I invite you to revisit chapter 2 HEAL and do some of the clearing exercises to release these negative emotions.

Shake What Your Mama Gave You

Exercise #10 Methods to Wake up Your 2nd Chakra

- If you're shy, start in the privacy of your own home.
- Practice dancing and moving in your own living room.
- Once you get more confident, venture out to a dance class.
- Belly dancing, salsa dancing, pole dancing are all great choices for waking up your 2nd chakra.
- Get a belly dancing hip coin scarf- these scarves are fabulous be cause they allow you to see, feel and hear the energy that your hips are producing. Plus they are really fun to wear.

Sexy Dance Class

I had the great privilege of teaching a sexy dance class at the Learning Annex several years ago. I had such a blast teaching this class. I also was amazed to discovered the amount of courage it took for most of the women to sign up for and attend this class.

Women from all walks of life showed up. Some were in their 20's, others in their 80's. They were different shapes, sizes and colors and they were all there for different reasons. There were women who wanted to learn how to dance for their partner, others who were single or divorced and some who were there just to support a friend. This was the case with Nancy.

The Doggie and the Boa

At the end of every class I would invite the women to go home and practice their new moves. The following week there were always splendid stories to share. I'll never forget one woman, Nancy. She was happily married for over 40 years and came to class in support of her best friend who was going through a divorce.

Nancy was fun, lively and a joy to have in class. That week I had prepared a sexy little routine for the women to practice that included a boa. I taught the women to enthusiastically swing the boa over their head then flip it between their legs with one hand and grab the other end from behind with the remaining hand. Then I showed them how to roll their hips seductively while moving the boa back and forth between their legs. This exercise was tons of fun, always got lots of laughs and really gave the women permission to drop their inhibitions and get their sexy on.

After class that night, Nancy headed home to give this new move a try on Bob, her husband of 40 years. She perched him on their bed and blindfolded him while she donned her sexy outfit and cued the music.

When Bob removed the blindfold, he nearly fell off the bed. He was stunned to see his conservative wife in her sexy lingerie, towing her boa, and touched that she went to all this effort just for him. Their family dog, a friendly golden retriever named Rocket was so intrigued that he parked himself on the floor, for a front row seat to the show.

As Nancy swung her stylish boa in the air and launched it between her legs, Rocket suddenly lunged for the boa. A tug of war ensued and Bob leapt up to assist her. Nancy, Bob and Rocket all tumbled to the floor in a pile of mass hysteria.

The following week, Nancy reported that they didn't stop laughing for hours and had the best sex they'd had in years. If you don't already know this, laughter is an incredible turn on and a wildly effective aphrodisiac.

Permission to Let Your Hair Down

Each week in class, I'd teach the women as much about releasing their emotional and sexual inhibitions, as I would dance moves. I remember one woman in particular, Maria, who walked into class wearing a white shirt buttoned all the up to her chin, glasses and her hair tightly wrapped up in two pig tail braids. She stood in the back of the classroom hesitant to do any of the movements.

I began working with her, encouraging her to just let go and feel the music. She started to respond so I placed my attention back on the class. When I glanced back at Maria, I was shocked at what I discovered. She had removed her button down, revealing a sexy t-shirt, whipped off her glasses and quite literally let her hair down. That astounding metamorphosis was ample reward, in and of itself. However, the following weekend I ran into Maria and her boyfriend and they both marveled at her transformation. Her Beloved chimed in saying how grateful he was to see her so relaxed and relishing in her feminine sex appeal. Maria's ability to giving herself permission to own her sensual and sexual feminine expression did wonders for their sex life as well.

Let's Talk About Sex

"THE AVERAGE AMERICAN HAS SEX 58 TIMES A YEAR—SO, ONCE A WEEK. IF YOU DOUBLE THAT, YOU REDUCE YOUR 'REAL AGE' BY ALMOST THREE YEARS."
–Dr. Memet Oz, Talk Show Host, Physician and Best Selling Author

Not only is sex deliciously fabulous and fun, it is also incredibly good for you, physically, mentally, emotionally and spiritually. The sexual union between two human beings is one of the greatest connections we can experience. Experts say that it is the closest thing to touching the Divine. So, let's talk about sex.

"I WANT TO BE RAVAGED OPEN TO GOD."
–*David Deida, Intimacy Expert and Author of "The Way of the Superior Man"*

Making love is an incredible way to move and heal your body for a multitude of reasons. On the physical level, it is one of the most delectable forms of exercise. You and your partner can enjoy your own private gym workout in the privacy of your own bedroom, bathroom, kitchen, living room, airplane bathroom… you get the idea.

Sex Helps Keep You Young

When you make love within the safety of a beautiful intimate collaborative relationship where both partners are being nourished, supported, respected and loved, the body is flooded with healing chemicals such as endorphins, oxytocin, testosterone and vasopressin. This has an incredible youthing effect for both men and women of all ages.

On the emotional, mental and spiritual level, those same chemicals that flood the body during sex also bond both people together, making a long-term relationship a sweet and beautiful possibility.

The bonding that occurs between intimate partners is incredibly valuable for each individual as well as for the wellbeing of the relationship. Individually, it assists the woman in feeling safe and cherished and the man in feeling respected and needed. These are the qualities that make a man or woman feel valued in the relationship. Lovemaking is also a wonderful expression of sexuality, sensuality, surrender and playfulness, which can be extraordinarily rich and healing for both partners.

"So, Are You Having A Lot of Sex These Days?"

There was a point in my life several years ago, where I made the conscious decision to stop dating for while. I needed to step back and do the work necessary to heal myself before entering into a new relationship.

Near the end of my dating hiatus, I went to my physician and she asked me point blank, "So are you having sex these days?" After I got over my initial, "That's really none of your business," primary reaction and then, "How in the world did she know I wasn't getting any?" secondary reaction, I inquired as to why she asked me that question.

She responded with a smile, "Sex is very, very important, especially for men and women over forty. It gets the juices flowing and helps keep everything lubricated and fresh." On an emotional level, it helps people feel alive and young again.

The sexual act itself when done with someone you are deeply connected with can also open you up to the highest spiritual realms. One of my favorite writers, David Deida speaks about being, "Ravaged open to God."

The relationship becomes a conduit in which both partners can gain greater access to the highest spiritual realms through the union of conscious, committed, tantric sex.

Taking it Tantric

Let's take it tantric for a minute. This word is used quite often, however, many people don't actually know what tantric sex is.

Tantra is the ancient art of lovemaking. It melds the spiritual and physical aspects of sexual union into a practice that opens both partners up to greater levels of intimacy and connection to each other and the Divine. Tantra is a beautiful ritual that can deepen any intimate relationship and spiritual practice.

There are many wonderful books and classes on the subject. I list several in the reference section located on my website, www.DrElizabeth.com.

With all this talk about sex, it is definitely time to grab our key and step through the next portal gateway to eternal radiance, LOVE.

Love

CHAPTER 5

Love

My fifth key to becoming undeniably radiant, beautiful, youthful and sexy is love.

You know, love is a funny thing. For such a simple four-letter word, it is a very loaded topic. There are a lot of misconceptions and preconceived ideas around this very potent word. We talk about it, want it, chase it, avoid it and even curse it but do we really know what true love is?

"IF YOU COULD ONLY LOVE ENOUGH, YOU COULD BE THE MOST POWERFUL PERSON IN THE WORLD."
–*Emmet Fox, Spiritual Teacher and Author of "The Golden Key"*

Love is the most powerful force in the Universe. It is the answer to every question and every challenge. Love is the richest of all my keys and the essence of the fountain of youth.

When I speak of love, I do not mean the romanticized, vacillating, swept away fantasy kind of unconscious love. I'm speaking about the energy that is the source of all that is.

I know in my heart that I have experienced the energy of unconditional love and I believe that each one of you have experienced it as well. It's the energy that brings tears to your eyes and angel bumps all over your body simply by being in its presence. It is the purest, most truthful word I know for God.

We recognize love immediately when we are in its presence because it is our true essence. Cut us open and you'll find love coursing through our veins and at the core of our DNA.

Looking into the eyes of a baby we recognize our own capacity to love unconditionally. With every smile they invite us to reclaim our inherent ability to love fully, freely and with no filters.

So, you might ask, "What does love have to do with skinny dipping in the fountain of youth?"

Well, actually, everything. Being able to swim in the energy of universal love is like having an all access pass to the fountain of youth for life.

What Makes Love So Powerful?

If each one of my keys opens a portal to the fountain of youth, unconditional love is like the wormhole that cuts through space and time and deposits us directly at the threshold of eternal radiance and youthfulness.

Love is another word for God, and God is another word for Light. When we love completely and freely, we literally fill our being with light. It is this light and radiance that gives us our eternal youthfulness. No matter what our chronological age, when we radiate Universal light and love, we become undeniably gorgeous and a magnet for all that our hearts most deeply desire.

There is Only Love and the Absence of Love, Which is Fear

The possibilities of what we can create with and in the energy field of love are endless when we begin to surrender our fears. As a species, we haven't even begun to tap into all the extraordinary miracles love provides.

When given half a chance, love can heal disease, mend hearts, fulfill dreams and even end wars.

"WHAT WOULD LOVE DO?"
–Dr. Michael Beckwith, Spiritual Teacher and Author of "Spiritual Liberation"

Anytime there is a conflict between individuals, groups of people or even countries for that matter, it is an invitation to infuse love into the situation. One of the most powerful questions I have learned to ask in any difficult situation is, "What would love do?"

The quality of our lives is determined by the quality of our thoughts and the questions we ask ourselves on a daily basis. When we ask ourselves, what would love do, it immediately shifts the energy of the circumstance.

This question invites me to pause and remember the truth; there is only love and the absence of love, which is fear. Just like there is only light, and the absence of light, which is darkness. Like a room that is dark, when we turn on the light, the darkness dissipates. The same thing holds true for fear. The moment we infuse love into any situation, the fear is dissolved.

"THE BEST AND MOST BEAUTIFUL THINGS IN THE WORLD CANNOT BE SEEN OR EVEN TOUCHED - THEY MUST BE FELT WITH THE HEART."
–Helen Keller, Political Activist, Humanitarian and Author of "Light in My Darkness"

If Love Really is the Answer, Why Don't We Choose It More Often?

For one thing, it takes courage to choose love. We live in a society that rewards being jaded, superficial and cool. Real love has no place in that artificial environment. Real love is messy. It is deep, genuine and completely authentic. Practicing unconditional love is like diving off the cliff into the ocean. It is terrifying but it is also the most exhilarating and extraordinary ride of your life once you surrender to it.

Most people, after their first encounter with heartbreak, swear that they will never be that vulnerable to the devastating pain of heartache again. So the walls go up… way up.

Because of the fear of being hurt, many people only permit themselves to know love intellectually from the logical mind. This approach allows them to safely view love from a tiny window in a fortress far above the risk of life's heartache.

The challenge with the brick wall strategy is that you can never truly give and receive love when you surround your heart with ironclad armor. Oh, you'll be somewhat successful in protecting yourself from being hurt, but you will completely obliterate any opportunity for mind blowing, heart opening, soul-stirring passionate love.

Here's the other thing about love. Since it is our true essence and the reason we came to this planet, when we don't express our deepest love, we can never truly be fulfilled. The longing we feel is like an insidious itch that can never be scratched. No amount of money, prestige, success, titles, fame or toys can fill the void of a heart that cannot give or receive authentic love.

To receive all that love has to give to you, you cannot merely use your five senses. You can't think your way into love. You must feel your way into it. One can only truly know love from the depth of a fully open heart.

Exercise #11 "Unconditional Love Meditation"

Find a place where you can get comfortable and will not be disturbed for a couple of minutes. Close your eyes and take a couple of long slow deep yoga breaths. Place your left hand on your heart and your right hand on your solar plexus (your tummy).

Place your attention and energy in your 6th chakra (your 3rd eye) in the center of your head. Keeping your energy in your 6th chakra, look down from within your body and see your 1st chakra at the base of your spine. Light it up like a starburst. Extend your grounding cord from your 1st chakra all the way down into the center of Mother Earth. (For a review on how to put your grounding cord down into the earth, see "Grounding Cord Meditation," Chapter 2 HEAL (page 49)

You can see your grounding cord as a steel beam, a beam of light, a strong oak tree, a string of pearls, a waterfall, a cable, whatever image works to ground you solidly into the earth.

Go ahead and ask your body to release whatever negative energy is ready to leave. You don't even need to know what that energy is. Your physical body will do this for you easily and naturally.

With your energy still in your 6th chakra, (at the center of your head), look up and see your 7th chakra (at the top of your head). Open up your 7th chakra and allow the sweet energy of the Universe to flow into you.

Simultaneously, invite the energy of Mother Earth to flow through your feet chakras (at the bottoms of your feet) and up into your body. Let the energy meet and swirl throughout your entire chest cavity.

Now with your attention and energy still in your 6th chakra, look down from within your body to your heart chakra in the center of your chest. Take a deep breath and as you inhale, light up your heart chakra like a starburst. As you exhale, feel deeply into the enormity of love energy that is in your heart chakra. Feel this deep, profound loving energy fill your entire chest and torso. Now see and feel this incredible love radiating out from your entire being. If you can't feel the love immediately, don't worry. Just continue to breathe and feel into the love that is present in your heart.

Remember that you are made of the same energy as the stars and the galaxies. Love is your essential nature. It is also your birthright. You cannot help but be love. Just relax and allow the love that is already within you to radiate naturally from you.

Continue to see from your 6th chakra (your 3rd eye) this extraordinary love energy emanating from your heart out into the world. Then see it circling back into you at the top of your head and the bottom of your feet. Feel this sweet loving life force fill you up and extend from your being in an infinite circle, ebbing and flowing like the waves of the ocean.

This experience may bring tears to your eyes. You may even have the urge to stop or suppress the flow of love because it feels so unfamiliar and overwhelming. Do not worry, hesitate or hold back, just surrender and allow this loving energy to continue to flow and fill you up.

I invite you to do this exercise everyday for twenty-one days. You will notice that each day it becomes easier to allow yourself to give and receive love in every area of your life.

You may also notice that you are beginning to feel more vulnerable, open, loving, caring, compassionate and kind to yourself, those around you and even strangers. That is one of the benefits of doing this exercise. As I mentioned at the beginning of this chapter, love is not a concept or an ideal, it is an experience. The more you give and receive love freely, the more you are filled up by its healing and rejuvenating energy.

Now that you've discovered this secret key, how can you bring more love into your life?

It All Starts With Self-Love

When talking about love, I find the best place to begin is with self-love. Everything we want, hope for and dream of emanates from self-love, self worth, self-esteem and self-respect. When we are able to love ourselves fully, we have the capacity to love others and infuse love into all situations.

How Can You Develop More Self-Love?

As I mentioned in chapter 2 HEAL, many people when faced with a question or challenge immediately turn their focus and attention out into the world for their answers. This is not where our guidance resides. There is nothing that the outer world can give you. Society will attempt to pull your attention so that you abandon your own power and inner knowing. Don't fall prey to these false advertisers. The truth is that you already have all the answers inside of you.

"LIKE LEARNING TO SWIM OR DANCE, YOU CAN'T JUST LEARN THE TECHNIQUE, YOU MUST DIVE IN THE WATER OR GET ON THE DANCE FLOOR AND ACTUALLY PRACTICE THE MOVES."
–*Gary Zukav, Spiritual Teacher and Best Selling Author*

I've been studying spirituality all my life and one of the things I have learned along the way is that it is not enough to master the concepts, you must put the information into practice in order to experience real change and transformation in your life. It is best if the practice is consistent in order to reap lasting rewards.

Here are some daily practices that will help you create more self-love:

- Forgiveness
- Meditation
- "Grounding Cord Meditation"
- Affirmative Prayer
- Service
- Daily Self Care
- Applying the principles in this book:
    - Choose to be willing to say yes
    - Heal and detox
    - Make healthy food choices
    - Incorporate exercise, stretching and movement into your life
    - Unconditional love of self and others
    - Daily Spiritual practice
    - Come together in community

Many of these practices are outlined in chapters 2 (HEAL), 3 (FOOD) and 4 (MOVE). I invite you to take time to revisit these chapters and practice these techniques. Incorporate them into your daily life and watch your self-love, self-worth and self-confidence blossom and flourish.

In Addition, Start Asking Questions

Take your questions into meditation and allow the answers to come to you. Write down any insights you may receive.

If something in your life is not working out the way you want, take time to go within and ask yourself, "Where am I not loving myself as much as I could?"

This exercise might sound like a simple solution but it is a very powerful practice. Remember, when facing a challenge, it is never about the other person, the outer circumstances or particular details of a challenge. The situation is always a mirror showing us where we can love others and ourselves more fully.

Ask yourself "What could I do to be more loving to myself?"

Examples might be things such as:

- Practice seeing yourself the way God/Love sees you, as perfect, whole and complete just as you are.
- Release and clear out negative energies of people, places and things that no longer resonate with your heightened levels of self-love, self-worth, self-respect and self-esteem.
- Whenever you are facing something that feels like it is too much for you to handle, remember you can always give it to God/Love/The Universe (whatever you call the Universal Presence) the angels and your guides and ask them to help you.

Next, ask yourself, "What relationships are draining me of my energy, life force or sense of self-love or self-worth?"

Write down the names that come to you. You may be surprised to discover that some of your closest relationships are actually draining you of your precious energy and life force.

Once you have spent time in silence asking these questions and listening for answers, come out of your meditative state and review the information downloaded to you during this exercise.

Ask your heart where you could begin to make changes based on these revelations. This is a powerful exercise. Your heart and spirit will contribute the messages you are searching for. Don't be afraid to make changes. Begin small if it feels too overwhelming to you and see how these shifts help you embrace more self-love, self-worth, self-confidence and self-respect.

"THE RULES OF TRANSCENDENCE INSIST THAT YOU WILL NOT ADVANCE EVEN ONE INCH CLOSER TO DIVINITY AS LONG AS YOU CLING TO EVEN ONE SEDUCTIVE THREAD OF BLAME. AS SMOKING IS TO THE LUNGS, SO IS RESENTMENT TO THE SOUL; EVEN ONE PUFF OF IT IS BAD FOR YOU."
–Elizabeth Gilbert, Inspirational Speaker and Best Selling Author of "Eat, Pray, Love"

Earlier I invited you to forgive for the sheer vanity of it. While that might sound a bit facetious, it is absolutely true. When your heart is filled with animosity and bitterness, you cannot give and receive love. As a result, no matter how physically attractive you might be, you will still look old, haggard and constricted. Real beauty cannot flow through a body that is filled with these negative emotions, it is impossible.

However, when you choose to forgive, the essence of who you truly are, love, can come rushing through you like a tidal wave of youthfulness. You will be gorgeous and wildly appealing to all those who cross your path.

Forgiveness is one activity that never goes out of style. No matter how much we pardon, there always more for us to exonerate. That's the nature of life and being human. The great part is, it certainly keeps us looking youthful.

Exercise #12 Forgiveness Practices

- Spend 5 minutes/day sending out thoughts of love and forgiveness to those who you feel have hurt you or whom you have harmed, intentionally or unintentionally.
- One of my teachers, Rev. Edwene Gaines, author of "The Four Spiritual Laws of Prosperity" shares this wonderful exercise:
- Think of someone you'd like to extend forgiveness to and write down on a piece of paper, "I _____ forgive _____ completely" 70 times a day for 7 days.
- Spend time every day in silence asking your heart and spirit, "Whom do I need to absolve today?" Include yourself in that meditation.
- Recite the "Ho'oponopono Hawaiian Forgiveness Prayer" daily and/or whenever you are faced with a challenging situation with anyone you are seeking peace, forgiveness and reconciliation.

Ho'oponopono Hawaiian Forgiveness Prayer

Recite out loud or to yourself the following phrase when seeking forgiveness, compassion and peace with someone with whom you are at odds:

"I'm Sorry, Forgive Me, Thank You, I Love You"

This is a very powerful healing prayer. When I first heard this invocation I thought, "Why am I saying I'm sorry? It is the other person who has caused me hurt and harm." However, what I learned through this practice is that, as I heal and clear any animosity in my own heart, I raise the vibration between the other person and myself, energetically healing all riffs between us.

I could write an entire book filled with astounding stories of how this prayer has worked in my own life. But, don't take my word for it... try it yourself and watch in amazement as you create your own miracles of forgiveness and love.

Learn to Love in the Face of What Appears to Be Unloving

True, authentic real love is the ability to unconditionally love even in the face of what appears to be unloving. It is recognizing that each human being is doing the best they can, given their circumstances and level of awareness. If they could do better, they would do better. This powerful realization allows us to view everyone with the eyes of compassion, kindness and understanding, no matter what the situation.

Practice Loving Without Expecting Anything in Return

Many of us love because we want something in return. This is not true love. Authentic love has no agenda; it just loves for the sheer joy of sharing its essential nature with the world.

When we love fully without expecting anything in return, something shocking happens. We begin to realize the mere practice of active unconditional loving showers us with more love, joy, peace, fulfillment and delight than we could have ever imagined.

This is an unbelievably stunning realization. Just give it a try and see for yourself how the practice of loving with no agenda floods your life with more love than you could have ever known.

We are all connected in an intricate web of energetic frequency. Even the smallest actions have powerful ramifications. When a butterfly flaps its wings in the Amazon, it can be felt in the North Pole. Make every thought you think and every action you take be one that is infused with the vibration of love and watch as exponentially greater amounts of love flow back to you.

Exercise #13 Practice Unconditional Love

- Today, make the decision to love with no agenda.

- Be aware and conscious of how and when you are dispensing your love.
- Begin to release any attachments to actions of "conditional love" as you observe them.
- Share a smile or a kind word with a stranger, or practice a simple generous act of kindness, such as letting someone go ahead of you on the freeway or at the grocery store.

These random acts of kindness flow out in concentric circles causing an exponential ripple effect of love and goodness that raises the vibrational frequency of the entire Universe and everything in it. Because of this fact, each loving action dramatically shifts our world in powerful and expansive ways.

Stop Caring What Others Think About You

This is your life. You have the power to choose what it is that you want to create, experience and love. When you begin to be true to yourself, the magic of love helps you create every single thing that your heart most deeply desires…everything.

Stop Putting External Circumstances Before Your Passion and Love for Who You Are and What You Truly Want

Here's a powerful reminder of the miracles that occur when you have the faith and courage to take a radical stand for your own self-love.

Taking a Stand for Radical Self Love

Suzanne is a very successful lawyer. She is also my beloved sister. For many years she was partner at a prestigious law firm. She went on to work as in-house counsel for a large corporation.

The company she was working for unexpectedly closed their doors one day and suddenly Suzanne found herself without a job. This was not an easy time for her. She had been used to a very lucrative career. She owned her home and had a great deal of financial responsibilities.

After months and months of discouraging rejections, a headhunter finally found her a job. Suzanne was tremendously grateful for this opportunity to work and bring in a steady income again.

Soon, however, her dream turned into a nightmare. The woman Suzanne worked directly under was verbally abusive. After months of attempting to talk to the woman and stand her ground, the situation came to a head. Suzanne had to make a very difficult decision. She had no new job lined up, however she knew in her heart that she could not allow this abuse to continue. It was having an effect on her health and wellbeing. She searched her heart and made the difficult decision to love herself enough to quit that job.

When she told me this story I was incredibly proud of her. It takes a great deal of self-love and courage to walk away from an abusive situation when it is attached to a paycheck that is necessary to meet your financial responsibilities. But she did it.

That bold action sent a message to the Universe that was undeniable. Within a couple of weeks, the headhunter called Suzanne with an offer for a better, higher paying job, in a much more peaceful and loving environment. In addition, Suzanne also manifested a magnificent loving intimate relationship with a wonderful man who is the love of her life. Suzanne and her Sweetheart, Walt, are now happily married and I've never seen her more radiant or beautiful.

When you stand for yourself and what it is that you truly want, the Universe rallies around you and brings you exactly what you desire. And sometimes, as in Suzanne's case, a good deal more than you even expected.

Stop Worrying About Being Hurt

Certainly this is much easier said than done. When the desire to express who you truly are becomes more important than being hurt or looking foolish, you will have the freedom and courage to open up and love with no limits.

Being Cracked Open to Love

I learned the power of being cracked open to love in 2005. I met a very handsome and charming man while I was salsa dancing with my friends. Antonio made a beeline for me immediately. At the end of the night he asked for my number and gave me his card.

When Antonio called, I agreed to go out with him. After several dates, he invited me to his home for dinner. When I arrived, Antonio walked down the stairs to greet me at his door. The moment our eyes met and he and touched my shoulder, a kaleidoscope of images scrolled past my eyes. In flashes of recognition, I was shown a beautiful past life that we shared together in great love. In that moment my heart opened to this man.

I had a lovely time with my Brazilian that night. I softened into his embraces and into his world. We began a wonderful courtship together.

I was not the least bit prepared for what happened next. Once he sufficiently enrolled my heart in this love affair, knowing full well that I was interested in being in a relationship, he proceeded to tell me that he's not really the monogamous type and that he wasn't interested in having a relationship with me.

Needless to say, I was absolutely heartbroken. I had connected with this man on a very deep and profound level. I had given my heart completely to Antonio. The heartache I experienced was so deep it felt like a heart attack. Intense pain radiated down my arms and hands and it was difficult for me to breathe. Those of you who have opened yourself up to love know that the physical pain of heartbreak is absolutely real.

As I drove my car home from Antonio's house speeding down the freeway in the pouring rain, tears filled my eyes. I cried so hard my eyes needed their own windshield wipers. My heart felt as if it was going to literally break open. And, in fact, that is exactly what it did.

Instead of getting angry with Antonio for his "seeming" betrayal, I took in every ounce of pain and heartache and asked Spirit to crack me open to unconditional love.

In that exact moment, I stopped feeling sorry for myself and just opened up my heart to Universal Love.

I asked to see myself for who I was "being" in that moment, a scared and wounded little girl who was just longing and searching for love and approval from a man and ultimately from my own father.

I also asked to see Antonio for who he was being, a scared little boy who himself had been deeply wounded in his own life. I opened up past the hurt, anger and betrayal and saw not only Antonio but all my past loves as frail wounded boys doing the best they could given their own levels of consciousness.

Then I saw my own father, as a very scared and wounded little boy, doing the best he could, given his circumstances and upbringing. Many images flashed upon my heart. I observed myself as a little girl on my father's lap. I witnessed him pushing me away because of his fear and inability to open fully to love. I watched him dole out miniscule amounts of conditioned love in return for my self-sacrificing vows of perfection and obedience. I witnessed how my own longing to have my affinity reflected back to me by my father as a young child resulted in abandoning my own life and dreams in order to seek his love and approval.

I felt profound levels of deep hurt, shame and abandonment. I didn't push it away, I moved into all of it. And just at the moment where I thought I couldn't take one more minute, my heart literally cracked open.

Such tremendous love and forgiveness for myself, my father and all my past loves poured forth. It was beyond anything I had ever experienced in my life. This rich soothing energy washed over my entire being and tears of surrender poured forth from my eyes so profusely I could hardly see.

In that moment I knew, as I traversed the chasm of heartache, I would never be the same. Now, this is not to say I would never experience heartache anymore, I certainly have. However I knew deep down in my soul that the fear and pain of heartbreak could never close my heart to love again. I knew that I had experienced authentic unconditional love.

My ability to release the anger, hurt and resentment of my heartache and move from victim consciousness to responsible participant with Antonio gave me another gift. It allowed us to become friends. This was a blessing beyond description. Although Antonio made a lousy boyfriend, he made a phenomenal friend. I could never have imagined the unconditional love and generosity I would experience from this man on a friendship level. When I decided to just show up and be unconditionally loving, friendship unveiled itself to be the most appropriate expression of that love for the two of us.

"LOVE IS JUST LOVE, AND THEN IT FINDS ITS MOST APPROPRIATE WAYS TO EXPRESS THAT LOVE."
–*Dr. Michael Beckwith, Spiritual Teacher and Author of "Spiritual Liberation"*

I don't believe that we "fall in" and "out" of love with people. We only show up "as" love, because there is only love. When we show up as love, we automatically find the perfect avenue to express that love.

I love my Mother and the way we express our love is as a beautiful mother and daughter relationship. I love my friends, and the way we express that love is in wonderful friendships.

Even though the love is expressed in different types of relationships, it is all still the same love. Therefore, our only task in life is to show up as love, and let the perfect expression of that love unfold naturally, easily and effortlessly.

Love is All That There is, Everything Else is an Illusion

Whenever someone chooses love, it's always going to end well, every time. I promise. So then, why would we ever choose anything other than love?

It is only fear that gets in the way of expressing authentic love. It also keeps us from just allowing love to be love. I see people all the time trying to put love into different categories, handing it out in different amounts to various people, measuring it out in small doses, trying to control it as a way to avoid getting hurt. But it never works.

Here's the secret. Once you allow yourself to dive off the cliff and be cracked open to love, you'll discover that the best, and only thing you can do is show up and BE LOVE. Show up as the full expression of love with everyone.

"YOU'VE GOTTA SING LIKE THERE'S NOBODY LISTENING, DANCE LIKE THERE'S NO-BODY WATCHING, LOVE LIKE YOU'LL NEVER BE HURT, AND LIVE LIKE IT'S HEAVEN ON EARTH."
–William Purkey, Professor, Education Expert and Author of "Becoming an Invitational Leader"

The freedom and exhilaration you'll receive from living your life this way is beyond what words can express. When you show up as the dispenser of love, you will be surrounded by and showered with so much adoration. The joy you'll experience is beyond what you could possibly imagine.

Here's the best part, when you allow your heart to be cracked open to love, you will look, feel and be younger, sexier, more radiant, more juicy, more beautiful and more appealing than ever. This is the reason uncondi-tional love is one of my top secrets to basking in the fountain of youth.

Wait for Real Love

"I NEVER STOPPED BELIEVING THERE COULD ONE DAY BE, BE A CHANCE FOR ME TO GET THE LOVE THAT I'D BEEN MISSING. SOMETIMES LOVE TAKES A LONG TIME. WAIT FOR LOVE, AND YOU'RE GOING TO GET YOUR CHANCE TO LOVE. WAIT FOR LOVE... WAIT FOR LOVE."
–Luther Vandross, Award Winning Singer, Songwriter and Record Producer

Everyday both men and women ask me how they can manifest the love of their life. For those of you dreaming of a beautiful intimate loving relationship, first of all, know that it is absolutely possible. Sometimes it can be very discouraging. Most couples today do not have relationships that we'd like to emulate.

The truth is that a real, deep and rich intimate relationship is achievable. I am very blessed to have many amazing couples who are my dear friends. I am grateful to them for modeling for me what a magnificent intimate loving relationship looks like.

My sweet friends, Ray Davis and Laurie Wilder are exquisite examples of a truly magnificent intimate loving relationship. Being in their presence is inspiring and their precious love for each other is palpable and contagious.

Conscious Loving is a Choice

During a recent interview I conducted with Ray and Laurie, I asked them to share one key to their success. Their answer touched me deeply. Going into their relationship, they both made the commitment to remain loving and keep their hearts open to each other at all times, even when they disagreed. Their commitment to each other, and their sacred union was greater than their need to be 'right' in any given situation.

If you're currently in a relationship, I invite you to incorporate this powerful practice into your lives.

"MARRIAGE IS A STRUCTURE FOR HEALING."
–*Dr. Harvelle Hendrix, Relationship Expert and Best Selling Author of "Getting the Love You Want"*

Most people, when they enter into an intimate relationship, do not view it as a conduit for healing and a place for their soul's expansion. And yet, that is exactly what it is. If you have an intimate partner who is also interested in healing, together you can grow, expand and share an extraordinary life together.

There is no more potent place for profound transformation than in the crucible of sacred intimate loving relationship. When you can look at intimate relationship as a place of evolution, you will give yourself and your beloved the gift of a lifetime.

If you're single, here are a few exercises you can do to help manifest the love of your life right now.

Exercise #14 Techniques for Manifesting an Intimate Loving Relationship

- Be on the look out for loving couples:
  - Make the intention to bring loving couples into your life.
  - Ask the Universe to bring you some wonderful examples of incredible loving relationships.
  - That can look like real life, movies, books, etc.
- Give thanks when you begin to see these examples because the Universe always gives more to a grateful heart.
- Celebrate it in others:
  - When you see a couple that radiates joy, love and happiness, send them a blessing.
  - If possible, tell them how incredible they are and what an inspiration they are to you.
  - People love to hear that they make a difference in other's lives, happy couples love to hear this.

- Connect with loving couples, their energy will bless you and help bring real love to you:
  - Ask these loving couples to see that vision for you. Where two or more come together in powerful intentionality, it exponentially increases the manifestation.
- Don't worry about being a third wheel:
  - Spend time with your friends who are in wonderful relationships
- Be your own beloved:
  - Spend time alone with yourself.
  - Don't wait for your beloved to arrive to do all the things you've always wanted to do. You never know, you might even meet your sweetheart in French class or raw cooking class.
  - Go to movies, dinner and/or the beach by yourself and enjoy the pleasure of your own company.
- Put yourself out there:
  - Sign up for dating sites. This sends a powerful message to the Universe that you're ready to date, even if you don't meet someone on the site.
- Act as if your beloved is already in your life.
  - For example, speak to them (as if they're already here) before you go to sleep at night.
  - Tell them about your day and about your dreams.
  - Talk about what you're going to do together.
  - Write them a love letter (with the intention that you will share it with them when they actually arrive in the flesh.).
- Let go of relationships that are close, but not exactly right:
  - When you hold onto a relationship that is almost right, you keep the one who is right from coming to you.
  - Continue to heal and grow while you're making yourself available to real love.
- Put it in plain view:
  - Create a vision board of exactly what you want.
  - Cut out pictures of couples who are engaging in loving activities that you wish to share with your beloved.
  - Yes, that means sexy pictures as well.

- ○ Make sure to use pictures and words that give you the experience of what it feels like to be with your sweetheart.
- ○ These simple practices rapidly magnetize the perfect love into your own life.

Keep your vision high and don't get discouraged. Remember it's darkest right before the dawn.

When you practice these exercises, I guarantee that you will bring an incredible loving relationship into your life. When you do, let me know and I'll celebrate it with you.

Now that you've been cracked open to love, grab your key and let's unlock the next portal gateway to the Fountain of Youth, SPIRIT.

Spirit

CHAPTER 6

Spirit

Enthusiasm = Spirituality = The Elixir of Youth

Enthusiasm is my secret elixir of youth. The word enthusiasm literally means, "In Spirit." One of the quickest ways I have found to swim in the sweet waters of the fountain of youth forever is to live your life in Spirit.

How Does Living Your Life in Spirit Help You Remain Youthful?

We are spiritual beings having a human experience. Our physical body is at the effect of the 3rd dimensional world (Earth). Therefore, it is subject to the passing of time.

However, as spirits, we are absolutely ageless, timeless and limitless in every capacity. When we step into the Divine (the Spirit realm), time stops and we literally do not age.

How Can You Step Out of Time and Into the Divine?

One of the quickest ways to step out of time and into the Divine is to do what you love in life with great passion and enthusiasm.

I see and experience the results of this practice first hand every time I am salsa dancing. Crowds of people gather to watch us dance at the Third Street Promenade in Santa Monica, California. They are captivated by the incredible joy, beauty and delight exuding from each dancer. I refer to this energy as "The JLF Factor" and it is what makes everyone look, feel and act years younger than their actual age.

Without a doubt, "The JLF Factor" (the Joy-Love-Fun Factor, Chapter 4 MOVE) is absolutely the X Factor of youthfulness. When we radiantly express our innate joy and love from our hearts through our physical bodies, we become undeniably gorgeous and forever youthful. "The JLF Factor" also helps us turn back the hands of time quicker than the best plastic surgeon's needle or knife ever could.

Have you ever noticed that when you do what you love, time stands still? This is because when we immerse ourselves in the universal vortex of love, we are lifted into the spiritual realm where time does not exist. Therefore our physical bodies do not age when we are in this higher dimension.

Think about it for a minute, spending a magical evening with your beloved flies by in the blink of an eye. Five hours seems like five minutes.

The opposite is true as well. Five minutes stuck in rush hour traffic on the freeway seems like an eternity.

The same principle holds true for your chosen divine employment. When you love what you do for a living, it doesn't even seem like work. Time is suspended and work feels like play.

Doing what you love also dramatically reduces the harmful stress levels in your body. The passion you feel when you express your unique gifts and talents floods your body with youth promoting endorphins.

Follow Your Heart's Desires

Sharing your gifts and talents as your divine employment is one of the greatest ways to skinny dip in the fountain of youth. Many people I speak with long to make a living doing what they love but have a great deal of trepidation about making the leap from a regular job that pays the bills to a fulfilling career that brings them joy.

Because of my own personal journey, I have tremendous passion for helping others discover and live their life's purpose. It's not always easy to follow your dreams. However, what I know for sure is that when you do, miracles occur to assist you, often times in very mystical and magical ways.

"A BIT OF ADVICE GIVEN TO A YOUNG NATIVE AMERICAN AT THE TIME OF HIS INITIATION: AS YOU GO THE WAY OF LIFE YOU WILL SEE A GREAT CHASM. JUMP... IT IS NOT AS WIDE AS YOU THINK."
–*Joseph Campbell, Mythology Expert and Author of "Hero with a Thousand Faces"*

Many people today are in jobs and professional careers that do not inspire them. Years ago, I was one of those people. And, like many people, I hadn't the faintest idea how to get from where I was, to where I wanted to be.

Back in 1985, that gap seemed so wide I could hardly imagine traversing it. As a young girl, I had been chosen to follow in my father's footsteps and become a doctor even though every cell in my body was screaming at me to follow my own destiny and life's purpose.

You see, my father loves being a physician. He is absolutely brilliant at and perfectly suited for his chosen profession. He recognized that I had the same quick mind and capacity for digesting voluminous amounts of information, so he determined that this would be the perfect career choice for his eldest daughter.

However, I had a very different destiny to fulfill. I had already been given glimpses of my soul's purpose as a child. Leaving my body, warping time and dropping into the abyss of the universe were commonplace for me growing up. As early as grade school, I loved writing inspirational speeches and sharing them with large audiences at the local University. I was enthralled with the concept of human potentiality, especially with regards to nutrition and exercise. These are the activities that lit my heart on fire.

Unfortunately my father didn't have the capacity to see who I was or the awareness to inquire as to what activities made my heart sing. Control and force were the methods he learned from his father and the only way, at that time, he knew how to parent. As a young child, I did not have the where- withal to stand in my power in the face of that kind of aggressive energy. So, I conceded to his forceful demands, figuring I'd pursue my own dreams afterwards. Little did I know at the time that this naïve game plan would be far more difficult to execute than I ever imagined.

After graduation, I suddenly recognized that I had dug a hole for myself so deep it would be almost impossible to climb out. I felt like I had placed my ladder of life against a building and climbed to the top, only to discover, with great dismay, that it was the wrong building. I believed that I had to climb back down, drag the ladder around with me as I searched for my building, prop it up against a new location and climb my way back up to the top. The entire idea seemed utterly daunting to me.

Little did I know, all I needed to do was sprout wings and fly to my life's purpose and destiny.

When I decided to leave my professional career, people said, "Are you crazy? Do you know how much money dentists make? What are you think- ing? You have it made, why rock the boat? You're throwing away years and years of grueling work and education." None of that mattered, compared to my sanity and the fulfillment of freely and fearlessly living my heart's desires.

I left my career with no idea what I would do, only a dream that I was here to share a piece of my heart and soul with the world in a way that only I could.

I found myself in various part time jobs, from sales girl to personal as- sistant. It was humbling and challenging but I was grateful that I no longer worked in a field that was so ill suited for me. I was thrilled that I had placed my life on a new trajectory. For the first time, since speaking on stage as a young girl, I felt hopeful.

Along the way, synchronicity stepped in. It always does once we decide to follow our heart's desires. Very serendipitously, without any prior training or experience in any of these occupations, I was given the opportunity to start a career as a professional skater at 37 years young, a television show host at 38, a dancer at 40, a journalist at 46 and a speaker at 50. What I have learned for sure is that if you are meant to be somewhere, nothing and no one can keep you from your destiny.

When I turned 50, people began asking me, "What do you do to stay so healthy and youthful?" I discovered that I had a wealth of knowledge to share with people from a lifetime of living healthy; body, mind, heart, soul and spirit. Soon, I found myself on stages passionately sharing my message. As I looked back upon my journey that led me here, I was amazed that everything I had done had perfectly prepared me for this exact moment.

As illogical as bouncing from doctor to dancer to TV host to professional skater, might seem, each one of these adventures perfectly prepared me for my current profession.

Today, after much forgiveness work for both my father and myself, I am grateful for the doctoral degree I earned. It is all part of my life's journey and destiny and assists me in helping others forgive, find their purpose and move forward in life with love. I also now understand that my father was only doing the best he could, given his own upbringing and level of awareness. Today I acknowledge him for the incredible growth and expansion he has also embraced in our journey together.

I am grateful for all of the challenges I went through along the way. They endow me with the grace, tenacity and wherewithal to encourage others to do the same.

No one can guide an individual to their heart's true desires better than someone who's lived a lifetime of doing it themselves. When you've walked through it yourself and come out the other side, you know without a shadow of a doubt that there's a light at the end of the tunnel and can guide anyone through that journey.

You know that, as you look across any chasm, you can jump because you've learned first hand that it's never as wide as you think.

If I Can Do It… So Can YOU

As you can see from my story, I can relate to anyone who is stuck in a career that does not suit them. When I was working as a dentist, I felt angry, stuck, bitter, frustrated, ashamed, unfulfilled, impatient and at times hopeless.

So, how can you sprout wings and fly to your life's destiny? Begin by having the courage to do what you love no matter what it might look like to the outside world, even if it doesn't make logical sense.

Exercise #15 How to Sprout Wings and Fly

Take a moment to decide what you'd like to create in your life. It could be as simple as a new outfit or as elaborate as your life's purpose.

Place a pen and a piece of paper, or a journal in front of you before you go into meditation.

Close your eyes and do "The Grounding Cord Meditation" outlined in chapter 2 HEAL (found on page 49). With your eyes still closed, place your attention on your heart chakra and feel it soften and open up.

Now ask your heart, what is it that you long to experience. As you begin to feel what it is that you want, if you find yourself going into the energy of not having it right now, just take a couple of long, slow deep yoga breaths and continue to place your attention on your heart chakra. You may begin to get flashes or pictures of what it is your heart is longing to experience.

For example, before I started dancing, when I did this exercise, I saw myself dancing as flashes or pictures in my 6th chakra, (3rd eye) in the center of my head. You may also hear or feel messages.

Don't worry if you don't see any images or get any messages right away. The important thing is that you enter into this meditative space with your heart and your soul wide open and trust that you'll receive whatever information is necessary for this particular portion of your journey.

Once you have completed the meditation, open your eyes and start to write down whatever information or pictures came to you. Don't censor what you receive, just continue to write for 3-5 minutes.

Do this exercise on a daily basis for the next twenty-one days. You will begin to get messages throughout your day and in your dreams. We never know when we're going to receive messages or where they're going to come from. It is not our concern. Our only task is to open up the channel between our higher selves and us and then welcome with gratitude each message that we receive.

When you receive a message, take action immediately. The logical mind may question the validity of the message or the significance of taking action. Don't fall prey to the lower levels of the logical mind. The more you honor the messages from your heart, the more effectively you'll be able to sprout wings and fly to each of your heart's deepest desires.

Search Out and Celebrate Others Who Have Sprouted Wings and Flown to Their Ideal Life's Work

In those times when my dreams felt very far away, seeing what was possible, through the example of others, was one of the things that helped keep me going. What struck me as incredible about those who stepped out of their comfort zone and shared their talents with the world is that each one of them listened to the whispers of guidance from the Divine.

When one person achieves their heart's desire, it is in the Universal vortex of creation. It then becomes possible for anyone else to manifest his or her dreams. If they can do it, so can YOU.

Following and Living Your Heart's Desires

"FOLLOW YOUR BLISS AND THE DOORS WILL OPEN WHERE THERE WOULD HAVE ONLY BEEN WALLS AND WHERE THEY WOULDN'T HAVE OPENED FOR ANYONE ELSE."
–Joseph Campbell, Mythology Expert and Author of "Hero with a Thousand Faces"

People often tell me that I'm a walking billboard advertisement for my business. They say, "Wow, you sure picked the perfect career."

The truth is, this profession, being an inspirational speaker, talk show host and author, picked me. I used to think it picked me when I turned 50. Upon further consideration, I decided that I began preparing for this career ever since I was a child.

But what I realize now is that I was born for this purpose. I actually came to this planet encoded with a particular set of unique gifts and talents that make me exquisitely qualified to teach this particular information to whoever wants to receive it.

The same thing holds true for you. Each of you came here with your own unique combination of talents to discover, cultivate and share. And the best part is that when each of us awakens to our purpose, together we will create a much more beautiful, peaceful and loving planet.

The Mosaic of Life

"THERE IS A VITALITY, A LIFE FORCE, AN ENERGY, A QUICKENING THAT IS TRANS-LATED THROUGH YOU INTO ACTION, AND BECAUSE THERE IS ONLY ONE OF YOU IN ALL OF TIME, THIS EXPRESSION IS UNIQUE. AND IF YOU BLOCK IT, IT WILL NEVER EXIST THROUGH ANY OTHER MEDIUM AND IT WILL BE LOST. THE WORLD WILL NOT HAVE IT. IT IS NOT YOUR BUSINESS TO DETERMINE HOW GOOD IT IS NOR HOW VALUABLE NOR HOW IT COMPARES WITH OTHER EXPRESSIONS. IT IS YOUR BUSINESS TO KEEP IT YOURS CLEARLY AND DIRECTLY, TO KEEP THE CHANNEL OPEN..."
–Martha Graham, Dancer, Choreographer and Artistic Visionary

For all of eternity, for all of time, there is only one YOU, with your divine, magnificent, unique combination of gifts and talents to share with the world. That makes you absolutely gorgeous. It also makes you vitally important to what I call, "The Mosaic of Life."

Each one of us is a brilliant and beautiful colored crystal of light and it is our purpose to shine our light as brightly as possible. Then, as we all glow together, we create this stunning "Mosaic of Life."

Just as sunlight summons a stain glass window to life, it is the light of the Divine, radiating through each one of us that beckons our souls to life. When each one of us brilliantly shines our unique gifts and talents, as only we can, the "Mosaic of Life" is complete.

Sometimes people question whether or not their gift is worthy of being shared. Even though it is often our joy to express our talents, remember, they are not ours; they belong to the world and must be shared for the betterment of humanity.

Many of you already know your gifts. Some of you are sharing them with the planet already either in your career or as a hobby. If you are not already sharing your gifts, here's an exercise to help you discover your purpose.

Exercise #16 Discovering Your Life's Purpose

If you are confused about what your life's passions are, look at what captured your attention growing up. Children, when left alone, will naturally gravitate towards the things they love to do and the things that they are good at. Both of those factors are necessary in choosing our life's purpose.

This exercise will require approximately 15 minutes to complete. Find a quiet and comfortable place where you will not be disturbed. Get out your journal or a piece of paper and a pen. Close your eyes and take a couple of long, slow, deep relaxing yoga breaths. Center yourself using "The Grounding Cord Meditation" outlined in Chapter 2 HEAL (page 49).

Once you feel grounded, ask yourself the following questions:

- What activities did you do as a child that captivated your attention for hours on end?
- What activities do you gravitate to now, when you have a free moment?
- What activities do you dream of doing or wish that you had the time to do?

As you ask yourself these questions, you can come out of meditation and write down the answers in your journal or piece of paper. Then take the next question into your meditation again.

If you have someone you trust, you can have them ask you the questions and they can write down the answers. Or you can record yourself while you're in meditation.

The main thing is to let go and trust what information you get in this meditation. Don't worry if it doesn't make logical sense; it may not.

Look for how your heart feels when you ask these questions and get your answers. If you start to get excited, get goose bumps (angel bumps), your heart starts beating more rapidly or you feel joyous, these are all signs that you are going in the right direction.

You may also get the sense that, "Oh no, this is too big for me." That's okay, just breathe and allow the vision to fully reveal itself to you. Often our life's purpose feels too big or too much for us to do. If we're given the vision, we are always given the means to fulfill it... always. Trust that.

Once you've gathered your answers:

- Make a play date, either alone or with friends or family and go participate in these activities.
- Leave the judgment behind. If you get guidance to go do something that seems unusual or different than what you thought, that's great, follow though with it. Sometimes our guidance stretches us past our comfort level and straight to our purpose.
- After you complete your play date, if you enjoyed yourself, go back into meditation and ask yourself the following questions:
  ○ What are my next steps regarding this activity?
  ○ How can I incorporate this activity into my career right now?
  ○ Whom should I talk to?

Continue this exercise until your purpose is fully revealed to you.

Remember, you can have more than just one gift to share. That's okay. Also, your passions may not be related. That doesn't mean you can't combine them into a unique business that can be very successful. Just follow your heart, not your head, and it will lead the way to the perfect expression of your gifts and talents.

Organizing the Crayons

My youngest sister, Christine used to play for hours and hours by herself. She would take the color crayons that my other sisters and brother used to make drawings and she would gather them all up and organize them in order of height and color. Once she was done with the crayons, she moved on to my mother's jewelry. She would line up each piece of jewelry according to size, shape, style and color. With each piece, she would lovingly pick it up, caress it, polish it, carefully place it down in its proper place and move onto the next one repeating the same actions.

When Christine graduated from college, guess where she got her first job? Nordstrom's jewelry department. She was the top sales girl there from day one. With tremendous love, she would present her customers with each lovely piece of jewelry, showing them how beautiful it was and how wonderful it would look on them.

She was so good at what she did that the Gucci timepiece representative hired her to be their sales rep. Again she quickly became the number one sales girl there. Other companies soon took notice and before long, Cartier timepieces became aware of her reputation. They offered her a wonderful job and soon she became the number one sales rep in the world for Cartier timepieces.

I share this story with you because the very same thing Christine did as a child, arranging and organizing beautiful things, led her to her divine right employment. She took her passion for beautiful things, her love of helping people, her desire for travel and glamour and parlayed that into an incredibly successful and rewarding career.

So what did you love to do as a child and what do you love to do now? They don't need to be related or make logical sense. Begin right now to mine the rich field of childhood pastimes and allow them to lead you straight to your life's divine purpose.

Don't Hoard Your Gifts for Someday

If you have a talent that you love sharing, don't wait to give it. Start offering it to people today. Don't wait for someone to invite you, sign you as a client or hire you. Passionately share those gifts with everyone you meet, and soon, opportunities to contribute your talents for pay will be knocking at your door.

Stop Saying I Need a J-O-B and Start Expressing From Your J.O.B., "Joy of Being"

If you are a singer, sing. Sing on the bus, sing at your place of employment, sing at the grocery store, and sing as you walk down the street. You never know who is in earshot of your angelic voice. If you sing for the sheer love of expressing your talents, you become undeniable. I promise you, someone will take notice and give you more opportunities to share your gifts on a larger and more lucrative scale.

This same practice holds true for any passionate gift you possess. If you're an accountant, start crunching numbers for people. If you're a clairvoyant or medical intuitive, start sharing your wisdom. If you're a movie producer, create a film. There are no limits to sharing our gifts except the ones we impose upon ourselves by our own fears. Allow your J.O.B., Joy of Being, to lead you to your next J-O-B.

Loving What You Do Until You Can Do What You Love

Some of you may be saying, "That all sounds great, but, as much as I'd love to do work that fulfills me, I can't just quit my job and run off and do what I really want to do. I have responsibilities and people who count on me. What can I do right now to reap the benefits of this youth promoting practice?"

That is an excellent question. And here's the answer. While you are designing ways to transition from your current job to one that is more suitable for the expression of your unique gifts, you can begin right now to love what you do.

That's right. Starting today, when you show up for work, you can make the decision to bring the energy of unconditional love to what you do. I can hear some of you saying, "That's crazy, how can I love what I'm doing when I hate my job?"

Here's a story that demonstrates the power of bringing love and forgiveness to what you do, even when it might be difficult or painful.

In 2004, I had a life altering conversation with one of my best friends and trusted confidants, Gail. We have been friends for many years and she had seen me try again and again to make one career idea after the next work, to no avail.

I experienced a level of success in various careers, however I hadn't yet found the opening to completely express my life's true purpose. I knew that energetically, something was holding me back from fully living my dream.

At the end of my rope, we had a conversation one day that changed the trajectory of my life for good. As Gail and I spoke about what was necessary for me to move forward, she looked me in the eyes and said, "You need to go back to dentistry, bless it, forgive yourself and your father and let it go with love." It was as if she punched me in the stomach. Those words literally knocked the wind right out of me. However, in that moment I recognized the truth, shook my head up and down and muttered, "You're right."

I took the next week, devoured several books and courses required to accumulate the 50 units of continuing education courses necessary to renew my state license. A friend from the gym, who heard I was a dentist, had been recruiting me for months to come work in his office. I called him up and had a job the following day.

Driving to work that morning took every ounce of courage I could muster. Besides being emotionally difficult, due to prior lower back injuries, dentistry was incredibly physically painful as well.

A transformational conversation with my dear friend and colleague, Dr. Joanne Coleman, driving to work one morning, shifted my perception and my experience.

She invited me to bring every ounce of love within me to this job. "Be a place of profound blessing to each patient you have the privilege to work on. Show up in service in that office and watch what miracles transpire," she said.

She was right. That day, I showed up in tremendous love and service to each one of my patients. I brought all the love that I had in my heart to this job. The patients felt it and benefited greatly from it.

A profound shift took place within me as well. Being a place of love in this office allowed me to open my heart, soften and forgive. I found a way to release the anger and resentment I had for my father, this profession and myself.

When you bring the energy of love to work, what happens is that you raise the vibrational frequency not only of that place of employment but also within yourself. Inevitably you're moved onto a more suitable and enjoyable work situation. And this is exactly what happened to me.

When I returned to dentistry, Spirit told me I would only be there for less than a year. Even though in the back of my mind, I knew that this situation was temporary, one day, as I was enthusiastically cashing a paycheck, I thought to myself, "Hmmm, maybe I could do this on a more permanent basis." No sooner did I embrace that thought, the Universe responded with a resounding, "No."

That "no" came in the form of a car accident one week later. The subsequent journey that ensued after the car accident brought me to my current profession as an inspirational speaker and author.

Sometimes our blessings are very cleverly disguised. At the time, I had no idea that car accident would bring me to this moment, writing this book, encouraging each of you to follow your heart's deepest desires, but I am very grateful that it did. I realize now that the particular experiences I had during that time were necessary to prepare me for my current divine employment.

As you can see from this story, bringing love to what I did brought me straight to doing what I love. It will do the same for you, if you are willing to apply this tool to your life.

Going to Work for God

After the car accident, I thought I'd be back at work within a couple days. Those days turned into weeks and those weeks turned into months. A year later, it became clear to me that the profession I trained years and years to do would no longer be an option for me. With no steady income, life became pretty daunting.

I applied for numerous employment positions as everything from cocktail waitress, to consultant, to server at a health food restaurant. I still remember gazing at the rejection letters, shaking my head in disbelief. After four (4) job interviews at a local health food restaurant for an $8/hour waitress job, I was told that I wasn't exactly what they were looking for.

Nothing seemed to open up for me. It was a very low point in my life. Then, one day, in meditation, I was given the message by Spirit to, "Go to work for God."

What Does it Look Like to Go to Work for God?

While I continued to look for gainful employment, I decided to go to work for the Universe. That "job" came in the form of service for my beloved Agape International Spiritual Center. At the time, the movie, "The Secret" had just been released and Agape was flooded with new visitors. I had the great pleasure of volunteering as an usher during service. I greeted people with open arms and an open heart. It was a very rewarding position and I adored my "job." Every Wednesday and every Sunday you'd find me at Agape welcoming people into our sacred center.

"DON'T TAKE THINGS PERSONALLY. NOTHING OTHERS DO IS BECAUSE OF YOU. WHAT OTHERS SAY AND DO IS A PROJECTION OF THEIR OWN REALITY, THEIR OWN

DREAM. WHEN YOU ARE IMMUNE TO THE OPINIONS AND ACTIONS OF OTHERS, YOU WON'T BE THE VICTIM OF NEEDLESS SUFFERING."
–Don Miguel Ruiz, Spiritual Teacher, Physician and Author of "The Four Agreements"

One of my favorite tasks as an usher was to pass out tissues. You might be wondering why I was passing out tissues. When someone comes to a spiritual center such as Agape or any place where their heart chakra is opened by tremendous amounts of unconditional love, it touches people very deeply and many times they cry. What I decided to do was send everyone a heartfelt hello each time I handed them a tissue. I would look them in the eyes with love and silently say in my heart, "I love you and it's going to be okay."

Since I was there every week I began seeing the same people. As I handed out tissues, I noticed that many individuals couldn't even look me in the eyes. They would take the tissue and immediately put their head back down. At first, the human part of me thought, "Well, I just smiled at them and told them that I loved them and they didn't even smile back." But Spirit just whispered in my ear, "Don't worry about it, just keep smiling, handing out tissues and loving them with all your heart." So that is exactly what I did.

Then one day, a woman came up to me and said, "I've been coming here for six months now. I see you every week and you always smile at me as you hand me a tissue. I couldn't smile back because I was in too much pain. My husband had just died and the only thing that kept me going was coming here to Agape. Even when I didn't feel like I had the strength to be here, I came anyway because I knew I would see you and you would smile at me, share your love and make me feel better. You are what got me through those first six months and I want to thank you from the bottom of my heart for your kindness."

I will never forget that day. It brings tears to my eyes just thinking about it. In that moment I realized the importance of always showing up in love and showering people with my love no matter whether or not they can return it.

As is always the case with service, when you share your love and generosity, you receive infinitely more in return, often times in very synchronistic ways.

I was no exception to this Universal Law. I didn't know how I would find my way to a new career opportunity, but I knew that service was the road that would take me there. And sure enough, quite serendipitously I met a wonderful teacher named Katherine Woodward Thomas and we became great friends. When she discovered what I had been through, my background as a doctor, my car accident and subsequent job challenges, she and her business partner, Claire Zammit invited me to attend a very prestigious conference as their guest. Many profound transformations occurred during that time that empowered and encouraged me to launch my business as an inspirational speaker.

Through Katherine, I met an incredibly gifted woman, clairvoyant healer, teacher and reader, Vicki Reiner. Completely out of the blue, Vicki called me up and shared that she had been guided by Spirit to offer me a scholarship to her clairvoyant program. The knowledge, wisdom and profound skill sets I have garnered in this course have absolutely transformed every single avenue of my life. Vicki, Katherine and Claire's generosities have truly been extraordinary blessings.

These are not the only gifts I received as a result of going to work for the Universe. Many other people showed up saying, "I was guided to gift you with this opportunity, this class, this book, this trip, etc." The level of generosity I experienced was beyond what words can convey. Truly, it was phenomenal and incredibly touching. I continue to be immensely grateful for all of these gifts and for all the angels who delivered them.

I have heard individuals say that they don't believe in giving things away for "free" because they feel the recipients never truly appreciate the gifts given to them.

I adamantly disagree, saying in response, "There is no such thing as 'free'." On a much grander scale, the Universe is always flowing in divine perfect energetic exchange. I gave love and support to those who needed it to assist in their soul's development and, in return, others gave to me exactly what I needed to further my own expansion. It's all a perfect dance and the more we can step into the Universal flow, the more we can be in this field of infinite abundant blessings.

Manifestation Exercise, "The Dance of the Divine Feminine and Sacred Masculine"

Another powerful exercise to assist you in becoming more radiant and youthful is an exercise I call, "The Dance of the Divine Feminine and Sacred Masculine."

These days, it seems as if everything is moving at warp speed. This is due, in part, to the fact that the vibrational frequency of the Universe is expanding. Sometimes it feels like somebody pushed the fast forward button on our lives. We don't even have time to accomplish our daily tasks, let alone the precious things we most want to do with our loved ones.

Because of this, I have created a manifestation exercise to help you generate much more in far less time with grace, ease and fun.

I call this exercise, "The Dance of the Divine Feminine and Sacred Masculine." This practice is a beautiful, delicate and perfectly balanced dance that occurs between two unique and opposite energies that reside within us, masculine and feminine.

As a woman who adores partner dancing, the concept of these two energies coming together in perfect harmony to assist in manifesting at warp speed is absolutely delicious to me.

What is the Divine Feminine Essence?

It is the energy of being, receiving, feeling, intuition and flowing. Feminine energy is all about insight. It is fluid, like the ocean and the wind, always moving, always in the flow of life.

What is the Sacred Masculine Essence?

It is the energy of doing, giving, thinking and logic. Masculine energy is all about action. It is solid and strong like a mountain and single minded in its focus.

So what does all of this have to do with manifesting more in less time and being more youthful? When these two energies work in harmony, with the Sacred Masculine being in service to the Divine Feminine, exponentially greater results occur.

Exercise #17 The Manifestation Exercise "The Dance of the Divine Feminine and Sacred Masculine"

The next time you have the opportunity to manifest something in your life, try this exercise and stand back in amazement at what you create at lightning speed.

Silence Before Action

Step One. Before you take action, sit down, take a moment and go into the essence of the Divine Feminine, which is your intuition. The way to access that space is through meditation. Close your eyes, take several long, slow, deep breaths. Apply "The Grounding Cord Meditation" as outlined in chapter 2 HEAL (page 49).

Once in this sacred space, ask yourself the following questions, "What are the first action steps I need to take? Who do I need to talk to? Where do I need to go? Where should I place my attention, energy and focus?" When you receive your answers, take the appropriate action.

This technique is based on the visioning technique developed by Dr. Michael Beckwith and the grounding cord exercise taught by Rev. Vicki Reiner.

Here's an Example of Manifesting at Warp Speed

For several years I lived alone in an apartment that I absolutely loved. It was right on the water by the boats in Marina del Rey. I liked my neighbors, enjoyed the building I lived in, and adored every day in this beautiful home I created for myself.

One day I got wind of a rumor that a large development company was buying our building, forcing everyone to relocate. Sure enough, a couple days later, I received my sixty-day notice on my front door. I couldn't believe it.

One by one, all my beloved neighbors moved out. It was heart breaking to see them go. I thought, "How in the world am I going to find a home that I like as much as this home, at a price that is within my budget?"

When the reality of the impending move hit me, I was guided to bring the question, "What action steps should I take?" into my meditation. I allowed my mind to be quiet and still and took slow, long, deep yoga breaths to center myself.

Shortly after I dove into this peaceful meditative state, I heard the voice of Spirit whisper in my heart and in my ear, "Ask Carol if she'd like to be your roommate."

Carol was a neighbor. We parked our cars next to each other for years and casually exchanged greetings when we saw each other in the parking garage. I always thought she was very nice but never thought of living together before my meditation that day.

I was a little bit surprised by the guidance given to me in my meditation. I enjoyed living by myself and hadn't entertained the option of sharing a home. But because this guidance was given to me while I was in the flow of the Divine Feminine energy, I heeded it.

After I came out of my meditation, I called Carol and asked, "What do you think about the idea of living together?" She was surprised by my question and said, "I was just thinking the same thing myself before you called."

This first part of the story demonstrates the decision to go into the flow of the Divine Feminine via meditation with a question or a dilemma and ask for Divine Guidance before taking any action.

Carol loved the idea of looking for a place together. We used the tool of visualization to create exactly what we wanted our new home to look and feel like. We were in agreement with what we were looking for in a home and it seemed like it would be a great fit for both of us. And, because we were coming together in one apartment, we could share the costs. We decided on a budget that would work for both of us and began looking.

The first place Carol and I visited met all the criteria we were looking for. But there was something about the energy of the people who worked at the rental office. Their behavior appeared inattentive, aggressive and uncooperative. We left that building in agreement that, even though it met our criteria, this was not the perfect home for us. The energy didn't match our energy.

Instead of randomly running around, looking at all of the other buildings in the marina, I decided to go back into meditation, this time with the question, "Where was the perfect place for Carol and I to live?" The answer I got thrilled me.

I was guided to check out the Dolphin Marina apartments. I had forgotten about this apartment complex. It was always one of my favorite buildings in the marina. I loved the name, Dolphin, and I loved the location. I also loved the look and feel of the building. On top of all of that, the woman who ran the rental office was a friend of mine who used to manage the building that

Carol and I lived in. What synchronicity. I called the complex and made an appointment to go see if they had any vacancies. Another synchronicity was that the leasing agent I spoke to on the phone at the Dolphin Marina Apartments, Kate, was the very same agent Carol happened to speak to when she was making her investigative calls.

It's very important when using this manifestation technique to look for synchronicities. They are Spirit's way of telling and showing you that you are on the right track. The antithesis is true as well. If things are not flowing and opening up, it could be a sign that it isn't right for you.

When Carol and I went to visit the building, we both commented on how kind the woman in the rental office was. It was a sign that this was a place that matched our energy. However, when Kate looked at her listings, she didn't have any apartments that met our original requirements. Instead of getting discouraged, I was guided to ask if she had any apartments in other areas of the building. Kate's eyes lit up. She said, "Oh yes, we just had an apartment come available right on the channel." Carol and I couldn't believe our luck. This was exactly what we were looking for. In fact, it was even better than what we were hoping to find.

Traversing the Eye of the Needle

I love this concept of traversing the eye of the needle. When an individual is ready for the next step in their transformational journey, they are given an opportunity to pass through the eye of the needle.

When we expand our consciousness, we are presented with an opportunity that shakes us to our core. An old outmoded way of thinking or being falls away, and we develop to a greater level. We must unfold to accommodate that new level of consciousness. I call this expansion, traversing the eye of the needle.

How we expand is very similar to water molecules. This makes perfect sense since we are composed predominantly of water.

If you apply a heightened vibration frequency to a water molecule, it amplifies in a very unique fashion. The water molecule will continue to vibrate faster and faster while maintaining the same shape and form. And then, suddenly, in one decisive moment, it pops open to a more expansive pattern. Each new pattern is more beautiful and exquisite than the previous pattern.

The same holds true for human beings. As life "rattles" us into an expanded level of awareness, we become more beautiful, more loving and more capable of holding and sharing Divine Light and Love. It is the challenges we face that simulate the pressure that is applied to the expanding water molecule in my example.

How the individual handles the challenge is what constitutes traversing the eye of the needle. The beauty of passing through the eye of the needle is that you're never the same. The expansion is permanent, there's no going back to a lower level of consciousness.

This next portion of Carol's and my story demonstrates traversing the eye of the needle. If we had just secured our dream apartment, picked up the keys and moved in, this would have been a great manifestation story. But, this was meant to be much more than just a great story it was destined to be a transformational journey.

Carol and I needed to be out of our old apartments by Nov. 9th. The dilemma was that our new dream apartment wasn't going to be ready until Nov. 17th. The people whose apartment we were moving into were going to move next door to the apartment that was being vacated at the end of October because it was a nicer apartment with a lovelier view. The turnover time was to take 17 days total. Somehow we needed to manifest a miracle so that we could move in on Nov. 9th instead of Nov. 17th.

It was time to go back into the energy of the Divine Feminine and seek the guidance from Spirit again. So I took my question, "What should we do about this gap in the timing?" into meditation. What I heard was a little bit unnerving. Spirit simply said, "Just trust that it'll all work out." Yikes, that's a tough pill to swallow when your back is against the wall, you need to move out and your new apartment isn't ready yet.

This is where the rubber meets the road. This is what constitutes the eye of the needle. One of my all time favorite books is "The Alchemist" by Paolo Coello. The moment Carol and I were facing was like the moment in the book, "The Alchemist" where the little boy must turn himself into the wind. How in the world do you turn yourself into the wind if you've never done it before? You must move into a level of surrender and trust in Spirit that you've never ever had to reach for before in your life.

Traversing the eye of the needle is like crossing the chasm where there is no bridge. This is the place where an individual crosses over into the level of absolute trust in the unseen Truth of Spirit. After you've done the dance of the Divine Feminine and Sacred Masculine, you've manifested what it is that you most deeply desire in miraculous and synchronistic ways, now it's time to cross the chasm.

So How Do You Cross the Chasm Where There is No Bridge?

This is the great secret to all of life. You step out on faith, belief and knowing. What I am about to share is what the wisest sages and shamans of all time have known and practiced.

Once you know in your heart of hearts that you've done all you can, you've merged intuitive guidance with divinely guided action, and you know in the core of your being that this is for you, you step out on faith.

When you decide to cross the chasm and you look across the gorge, you notice that there is no bridge. As you take the subsequent step onto what feels like thin air, at that exact moment, the next wood plank of the rickety bridge appears directly under your foot. If you didn't see it with your own eyes, you would never have believed it.

I love that image. It reminds me of that amazing scene from the movie,

"Frozen" where Elsa sings, "Let it Go." As she lets go of her fears and begins to own and express her unique gifts, she literally creates a bridge of ice out of thin air that carries her across the gorge to the mountain top.

This is where Carol and I were standing. Across the chasm, through the eye of the needle, was our new home and new life. The only way to get there was absolute trust in something unseen and unknown which was greater than us.

Oh, we still made some back-up plans. We called storage companies to see if we could put all of our belongings in pods for those 8 days. We called friends to see if we could bring our overnight suitcase and sleep on their couch. But deep inside we knew that something was going to open up to allow this move to happen with grace and ease. We just didn't have a clue at that moment what it was going to be.

Then, on October 31st I received a call from Kate at the Dolphin apartment rental office. It's absolutely amazing to me how you always know on such a deep intuitive level what is about to happen before it actually occurs. When I answered the phone, Kate said, "Something's happened." Even though my logical mind was on the verge of protesting, "Oh no, something's wrong, we're going to lose the apartment," somehow, the greater part of me instantly knew that our miracle was on the other end of this phone call. Kate told me that the people who were going to move next door decided not to move and that we could move into the nicer apartment on Nov. 9th.

I just sat there, staring at the phone, hardly able to believe what I was hearing. Carol and I never even thought our solution could have come in the form of moving into the better apartment with the nicer view so as to meet our deadline. It was beyond what we ever dreamed possible.

Kate invited us to come look at our new apartment that day. Carol and I looked at each other, stunned at our good fortune. In those 10 days before October 31st when our solution came, we just kept putting one foot in front of the other across that chasm, building our bridge on faith and trust.

But it doesn't end there. In my meditations, I had been asking Spirit to send me the perfect person to help edit my book and manage my career. Before moving in together, Carol and I spoke briefly about my business. She even attended some of my seminars.

A couple of days before we moved in together, she asked me if I could help her manifest a stronger, healthier physical body. I told her that it would be my pleasure. I agreed to coach her on a healthy living foods lifestyle and she committed to that journey with me.

Then she asked to see my book manuscript. I informed her that it wasn't done yet and she looked me straight in the eyes and said, "You know I'm an editor." I nearly fainted. The synchronicity was mind-boggling.

Carol was my exact target market. She was opening up to her spiritual essence and longed to become healthier. I had been asking for the perfect editor and Spirit delivered one right to my new dream home's front door in the form of the perfect roommate. It was an absolute match made in heaven.

At the time of writing this chapter, Carol and I have been in our new home for over two years. We still give thanks every day for this wonderful blessing. So many miracles have occurred since moving into our new home. Carol manifested a fabulous new job at a great company, working with wonderful people. And I have completed my first book.

When you apply these manifesting principles and have the courage to traverse the eye of the needle, the possibilities of what you can create in your life are endless.

Once you've tapped into your spirit, it's time to come together in collaboration to reap the benefits of COMMUNITY.

Community

CHAPTER 7

Community

"GARDENS CREATE COMMUNITY. THE EARTH IS MY CANVAS AND MY GARDEN IS A TOOL FOR THE TRANSFORMATION OF MY COMMUNITY."
–Ron Finley, Fashion Designer, "Renegade Gardener" and Humanitarian

Human beings thrive in community. What we want most in life is to be loved and to belong. And yet, many people spend most of their time alone. There is a lack of real authentic heart-to-heart, soul-to-soul human connection today. It is not unusual for someone to drive to and from work by themselves, spend all day in a little cubicle, eat unaccompanied, go to sleep alone, wake up and do it all over again.

With the evolution of technology, even when people come together, they can still be isolated. I often see couples walking down the street, side by side talking on their cell phone to another individual, completely oblivious to the precious opportunity for human connection that is right in front of them.

The family structure often lacks connection as well. Recently I saw a family driving down the freeway in a SUV, with one child playing a video game, one watching a movie, mom on the phone in the passenger seat and dad driving silently down the freeway.

However, this doesn't have to be the case. Instead of allowing technology to separate us, we can now utilize it to connect to one another across the globe. With the advent of the Internet, someone in New York City can connect virtually face to face with someone in a small village in Ghana, West Africa.

Authentic connection in community is vital to the expression of one's soul and the health of their heart, mind, body and spirit. Even if you enjoy time alone, everyone needs to connect with other human beings.

If you look back at history, tribal societies lived in powerful communities and flourished. They ate together, celebrated together, laughed together, grieved and healed together. And because of this, they thrived together.

Why Are So Many People Isolated?

There are many reasons why people are isolated from one another. There are physical factors such as the emergence of sprawling metropolises such as Los Angeles. There are also emotional factors such as protection from getting hurt, and an ever-increasing lack of care and concern for those around us whom we are not familiar with. Life moves so quickly. Most people are just too busy trying to get by and make things happen in their own little world to reach out to people outside of their inner circle.

Fear also plays a large role in the increased levels of isolation. People keep their distance from one another out of a sense of self-preservation. Fear separates and love unites. It is only fear of being hurt, judged, rejected, feeling out of place or wrong that keeps people from reaching out to connect with others.

Now, I'm not talking about personal alone time or sacred time to connect with the Universe in meditation, prayer and contemplation. I'm talking about a severe lack of heart-to-heart human connection. When we come together with other like-minded people in sweet fellowship we create conscious communities. These communities are incredibly healing.

I love the idea of conscious community. Magic happens in this arena. We have the capacity to bring out the best in one another and ourselves in conscious community.

What is conscious community? It is when people deliberately come together to share with one another.

What do they share? They share everything from ideas and solutions to encouragement and love.

In the mathematics of humanity, one plus one equals infinity. Community offers solutions to life's greatest challenges by coming together in collaboration, cooperation and co-creation.

Take nutrition for example. Here's a powerful story about one man, an artist, who turned the barren patches of dirt that line the streets of South Central Los Angeles into beautiful gardens of hope, health, education and inspiration.

I discovered Ron Finley quite synchronistically. A friend of mine on Facebook posted a video of Ron speaking at a recent TED Talk. Her jubilant enthusiasm for this man and his vision inspired me to watch the video. I am so grateful for her recommendation.

Ron Finley caught a powerful vision for his community. As he looked around his neighborhood he realized that the street corners were lined with liquor stores and fast food restaurants. He noticed that nowhere in this neighborhood was healthy, organic fresh produce available. He personally had to drive 45 minutes, each way, just to procure whole foods for himself. Everywhere he looked, he saw the out-picturing of junk food consumption in the physical bodies of his neighbors. Obesity was rampant. People suffered from completely curable and preventable diseases such as diabetes because proper education and nutrition weren't accessible.

He also noticed that right under his nose were barren plots of land that were just waiting to be transformed into gardens. So that is exactly what he did. Intrigued at the unusual vegetation popping up in their neighborhood, people began asking Ron what he was growing. Ron's garden offered a way for neighbors to reach out and connect as well as nourish and educate.

He enlisted the youth of his community to help him grow and tend to these delicious gardens and inspired their interest in healthy living.

Kids Who Plant Kale, Eat Kale

Ron taught the kids about the value of these nutrient dense veggies and soon they began replacing junk food with living food. Because of his enormous generosity of heart and spirit, he offered this organic, healthy produce to those who needed it.

One evening, around 10:30 pm Ron saw a young mother and daughter cautiously picking some of his organic produce. When he ventured out of his home to say hi, he noticed the shame this young woman felt for picking his produce. He quickly put her at ease, assuring her that he planted the produce there on the street to give his neighbors access to healthy living nourishment and invited her to take whatever she needed.

Ron created co-ops and employed the people in his neighborhood to work at these establishments, giving them a job, self-respect and a new purpose for living. This man is making a tremendous difference in the lives of so many people. He is giving them the keys to health, wealth and well being and showing them a better way.

This is a brilliant example of the extraordinary benefits of community. When people come together magic and miracles happen.

"But Dr. Elizabeth, What if I Don't Have a Community?"

What if you don't feel like you belong to a community? I hear this often from people when I speak at events or work with clients.

Some people are fortunate enough to be born into a family or community that they love. There is a deep connection between them and they wish to spend quality time together. To others, this sounds like a death sentence.

If you do not feel a strong bond with your blood family and birth community, don't fret. There are many things you can do to foster community in your life. Rest assured you can find your own tribe. Your passions and interests are the clues that lead the way.

Exercise #18 How to Find Your Tribe

First ask yourself:

- What are my interests?
- What am I passionate about?
- What do I love to do?
- How do I love to spend my free time?

If you don't know what you're passionate about, I invite you to review Exercise #1 (page 12), Exercise #15 (page 162) and Exercise #16 (page 165). All three of these exercises will help you discover what lights you up inside and gives you great joy. I recommend that you revisit these exercises before proceeding.

If you can answer these four questions, get out a piece of paper and a pen and write them down. I suggest that you close your eyes before beginning this exercise and take a couple of slow deep yoga breaths. Then place your grounding cord down into Mother Earth (as described in chapter 2 HEAL, page 49).

Ask yourself these questions while in this deep meditative state. You'll be amazed at what your soul is longing to share with you once you get quiet enough to listen.

Once you come out of your meditative state, place the pen on your paper and start journaling. Don't edit or judge what you are writing, just continue to let the answers flow out of your heart and onto the paper.

Give yourself 3-5 minutes to finish your free flow writing. Then take a peak at the list you have created. You may be very surprised at the things your spirit and heart are longing to do that your logical mind has been censoring. Don't say no to any of the ideas you wrote down on the page. Just allow them to land on your heart and sink in.

Over the course of the next couple of days, ask yourself this question:

What if I allowed myself the pleasure of _____?
(Fill in the blank with whatever activity came through in the exercise)

For example:

- What if I allowed myself to travel overseas?
- What if I allowed myself to start a business?
- What if I allowed myself to go back to school?
- What if I allowed myself to learn how to dance?
- What if I allowed myself to take a painting class?
- What if I allowed myself to learn a new language?
- What if I allowed myself to train for and run a 10K race?
- What if I allowed myself to take a raw food cooking class?
- What if I allowed myself to learn how to play an instrument?
- What if I allowed myself to start writing the book I always dreamed of creating?
- What if I allowed myself to open up my heart and share who I am a little bit more?
- What if I allowed myself to learn to surf, ski, play basketball, etc? (fill in the blank with your particular physical expression)

Just begin to open up to the possibility of incorporating these activities into your life.

Next, go to the Internet and Google your activity. For example, since I have a passion for salsa dancing, I would Google "Salsa Dancing in Los Angeles."

Check out what kind of community organizations such as "Meet Up" are offered in your neighborhood.

For those of you who are not familiar with "Meet Up" it is a website that's all about neighbors getting together to learn something, do something, share something. Their website is www.meetup.com.

Some people love to venture out on their own. Others prefer the company of friends. If you are the latter, ask a friend to join you. Either way, just get started. Once you dive in, you'll be amazed at the amount of joy community can bring you.

Here's an example of the communities in my life and how I discovered them. I share this information as an example of how you can create community in your own life.

For me, personally I have four amazing communities to which I belong. Each one of these communities is rooted in one of my passions.

For example, I love to workout. One of my communities is Gold's Gym in Venice, California. You can find me there pretty much every day of the week at 8am (except Sunday morning, when I'm at one of my other communities, Agape). I have been a member of this gym since 1995 and it is one of my homes away from home. Walking into the gym is like taking in a breath of fresh air. I am showered with love and offered the opportunity to see my sweet friends every morning. Visiting the gym has become as important to the health of my heart as it is to wellbeing of my physical body. I have met some incredible people over the years at my gym.

My next community is my beloved spiritual community, Agape. I have been an active member since 2000. I have learned profound spiritual lessons and have incredibly deep and rich friendships with the people of this community. When I walk into Agape, it is like coming home. The sweetness I feel enriches my life beyond what words can convey. I can't imagine my life without this beautiful place in it.

My third community is my salsa dancing community. As award winning singer/songwriter/prodcuer, Charlie Wilson sings, "Oooh Wee," how I adore this community. How could you not love a place where handsome men sweep you up in their big strong arms and whisk you around the dance floor in a passionate embrace? To me, salsa dancing is like making love on the dance floor. Where else, besides possibly the tango dance floor, can you experience such sensuality, sexuality and passion with your clothes on in a PG fashion? It is delicious and incredibly healing.

My fourth community is my raw food community. I am so grateful to have been welcomed with open arms into this healthy, vibrant and glowing group of people. We share a deep passion for foods that nourish us from the inside out and love sharing our knowledge of whole living foods with others who are interested in getting their raw food glow on.

Each one of my communities reflects one of my interests and passions. Coming together in community gives you a double dipping into the fountain of youth. You give yourself the opportunity to do what you love, which in turn allows you to glow from the inside out. Then, as you come together with other people who share your interests, you get the opportunity to dive once more into the fountain and receive the youthful benefits of being around others who share your passions.

Sometimes we find our communities effortlessly, as I did with my salsa, gym and raw food communities. Other times, it requires a bit of surrendering to get there.

It Took a Crowbar to Pry Me Out of My Own Way

To say I had a little resistance around going to Agape would be the understatement of the century. I was raised in a very strict Catholic household.

My father went to church everyday and insisted that we joined him.

Even as a very young child, I never resonated with religious rules and dogma. I've always had the awareness that religions separate and spiritually unites. I never understood how people could kill each other over whose God was better. It makes absolutely no sense to me.

Once I became an adult, I found my own way to express my spirit out in nature. So when a girlfriend invited me to attend her "church" I replied with a very gracious yet adamant, "Thanks, but no thanks."

But Spirit always has a better plan, and, as fate would have it, this friend did a favor for me. When I asked her how I could reciprocate, she quietly said, "Come to Agape with me." I shook my head and implored, "Anything but that, please." She just held firm to her request.

It was a Wednesday evening in mid October. Still trying to wiggle out of this commitment I said, "Isn't there something else I could contribute to you?" Exasperated, she just replied, "Do what you want Elizabeth, I'll be attending service this evening."

At that moment, I was overcome with a strange feeling inside of me. I closed my eyes and simply took a deep breath. In that breath, I heard the whisper of Spirit say, "Just go. Trust me." It took every ounce of strength to muster up an affirmative answer.

What I know now is that in that moment, I had to release the painful wounds from my strict religious upbringing. I had to let go of the patriarchal control, harsh rules, regulations and rigidity that nearly strangled the life out of my free spirit growing up. I had to forgive and let go of all of it from this lifetime and from many lifetimes past. And I knew it in that moment.

"REMEMBER ONE RULE OF THUMB: THE MORE SCARED WE ARE OF A WORK OR CALLING, THE MORE SURE WE CAN BE THAT WE HAVE TO DO IT."
–*Steve Pressfield, Novelist, Screenwriter and Author of "The War of Art"*

This wasn't just about going to Agape. It was about stepping into a brand new life. Somehow, deep in my intuitive awareness, I knew this and I was scared.

But I did it. And it became one of the most important and profound decisions of my life. I got my career, my joy of dance, my dedication to service, my spiritual growth and development and some of the most precious friends in my life from Agape.

As I showed up that Wednesday evening at 6:30 and sat next to my friend, another prophetic experience occurred. The moment I sat down in my chair and looked up at the stage, I saw a vision of a brilliant and inspiring dance performance. All the dancers were in white and I was high above my dance partner's head spinning in an intricate aerial lift.

That exact vision came to fruition on Easter Sunday, 2005. It was the very first time I danced on stage with the dance ministry called Movement of Agape.

I share this story with you as a reminder to remain open to the miraculous ways you may be guided to your communities. Recognize that the resistance you feel is actually an invitation to let go of old wounds that are standing in the way of your future greatness. I am not saying that it is easy, it certainly wasn't for me, but it was definitely worth it. And, as my own life's experiences have shown, it always is.

Global Communities

Once you awaken individually, you have the opportunity to come together with other awakened souls and make a difference collectively. Because of the synergistic effect community creates, together we can do much more than we could on our own.

There are many challenges facing the world right now. If you have a dream and passion to make a difference but you don't know where to begin, start by talking about it. You never know who else might share your vision. You can make a difference in your family, your local community, your state, country or globally. Begin today with one small action step.

Many people get overwhelmed because they think that the problem is too big and say, "What can one person do to make a difference?" But just one small action can make all the difference in the world.

The Little Boy and the Starfish

There was a little boy walking along the ocean one day. It was low tide and thousands of starfish were washed up on shore. One by one the little boy began placing the starfish back in the water.

An old man walked up to him and said, "Why are you bothering to toss those starfish back in the water? There are thousands, and you'll never be able to return them all to the ocean. You can't possibly make a difference." The little boy replied as he gently placed a starfish back in the water, "I just made a huge difference to this one." –*Author unknown*

Sometimes all it takes to make a difference is to take the first step. Here are some ways you can begin to be a contribution in your communities:

- Share your dream with others
- Be willing to take the first step
- Giving loves company so serve together
- Make it social and fun

Showing up in service is an incredible way to swim in the sweet waters of the fountain of youth. Nothing youths you quite like service. Giving to others is one of the most magnificent gifts you can give yourself. Once you get that concept, you will always remain forever youthful.

A perfect example of someone who retained her youthfulness by giving service is Audrey Hepburn. She gave of her heart and soul and absolutely glowed with grace, beauty and radiance her entire life.

The Incredible Power of Good... Good... Good Vibrations

A couple of years ago I had the great privilege of hearing the late Dr. David Hawkins, author of "Power vs. Force" speak at a conference. The level of light and love that this man emitted was stunning. What struck me most powerfully was his ability to find and express beauty, unconditional love and authentic joy in everything and everyone. During his talk he laughed often and easily as he shared his wisdom and uplifted the entire room with his light.

A remarkable physician who artfully merged the studies of science and spirituality, Dr. Hawkins created "The Map of Consciousness." Utilizing muscle testing, he was able to determine and chart the levels of awareness of people, places, circumstances and events.

So What Does this Have to do With Looking and Feeling Younger, More Radiant and Beautiful?

Well, everything, actually. What Dr. David Hawkins determined is that the energies of hate, greed, prejudice, competition, shame, guilt, anger, etc., vibrate at a very low frequency. A person engaged in such expressions appears harsh, worn, old and lifeless no matter how physically attractive they might be.

On the other hand, the energies of love, joy, kindness, peace, generosity, compassion, light, etc., vibrate at a very high frequency. An individual engaged in these expressions appears vibrant, radiant, youthful and alive, regardless of their age or physical appearance.

While speaking to a room filled with one thousand highly conscious people, Dr. David Hawkins posed the following question to the scientifically proven technique of muscle testing. "This group of one thousand highly conscious people has the power to counterbalance the negative energy of how many people?"

His response shocked and inspired me. Dr. Hawkins was able to determine that one thousand highly conscious people are able to counter balance the negative energy of 65 million people!

If one thousand highly conscious people can counter balance the negative energy of 65 million people, then it would only take one hundred ten thousand awakened souls to counter balance the negative energy of the entire planet. That means when one hundred ten thousand highly conscious people collectively come together, we can potentially reach the global tipping point.

What is a Tipping Point?

A TIPPING POINT IS, "THAT MAGIC MOMENT WHEN AN IDEA, TREND OR SOCIAL BEHAVIOR CROSSES A THRESHOLD, TIPS AND SPREADS LIKE WILDFIRE."
–Malcolm Gladwell, Journalist and Best Selling Author of "The Tipping Point"

As Dr. David Hawkins demonstrated, there is exponentially more power in the high vibration of love, joy, generosity, kindness and light than there is in low vibration frequencies.

As more and more people awaken, they begin to vibrate at higher levels of consciousness. When we come together in elevated frequencies, we can create miracles. Here's an example of one such miracle.

It Would Take 2 Feet of Snow in July to Reduce Crime

In Washington DC, one of the highest crime capitals in the world, a scientific study was conducted by Quantum Physicist, Dr. John Hagelin. He gathered together four thousand experienced meditation experts. The goal of the meditators was to create an energetic environment that increased coherence and reduced stress by raising the vibrational frequency through meditation. Dr. Hagelin believed that meditating for long periods of time during this eight-week study would reduce the crime rate by over 20%.

The chief of police in Washington DC said that it would take 2 feet of snow in July to reduce crime by 20% in DC. Not only did this study prove the skeptical police chief wrong, before the end of the experiment, the entire police department became a collaborator of the study. Indeed, as a result of the energetic calming influence of the meditation group, the rate of violent crimes decreased by 23 % during that eight-week period.

Think about this for a minute. If four thousand highly conscious light workers can lower crime in the crime capital of the world by 23%, anything is possible. Armed with this capacity to shift energy from violence to peace and low-level frequency to high, we can use these practices to solve every one of the challenges facing our planet and humanity right now. We have at our fingertips the solutions to every one of the problems facing our world. The answers are within our own grasp and the tools are right here in this book. It starts with each one of us individually.

"SO WHAT IS THE SOLUTION? WE CAN LOVE. REAL LOVE. TRUE LOVE. BOUNDLESS LOVE. FROM THE MOMENT WE WAKE UP TIL THE MOMENT WE GO TO BED, PERFORMING ACTS OF KINDESS BECAUSE THAT IS CONTAGIOUS. ... INSTEAD OF TRYING TO CHANGE OTHERS WE CAN CHANGE OURSELVES, WE CAN CHANGE OUR HEARTS.... AND ONCE WE TRULY LOVE, WE CAN MEET ANGER WITH SYMPATHY, HATRED WITH COMPASSION, CRUELTY WITH KINDNESS. LOVE IS THE MOST POWERFUL WEAPON ON THE FACE OF THE EARTH."
–Prince Ea, aka Richard Williams, Artist, Musician and Social Activist

I recently discovered a video on the Internet created by a very powerful social activist and artist, Prince EA, aka Richard Williams. I was blown away by his heart, talent and dedication to making a difference in the world.

After watching his inspiring video, "Why I think *this* world should end," I had a thought. There are over 50 million people who have viewed this video. What if just five hundred of those individuals made the decision to practice the solutions Prince Ea is suggesting in his video and I am inviting you to embrace in this book? Based on what Dr. David Hawkins shared regarding the global tipping point, We could raise the frequency of every major city in the United States.

If five thousand joined in, we could raise the vibrational frequency of most of the cities in Europe. And if just one hundred ten thousand rallied with us, we would engage in the tipping point, creating an exponential ripple effect of goodness that would cirlce the globe, permanently shifting the world for the better. It is simple, not necessarily easy, but definitely worth it. I'm in... will you join us?

"BE THE CHANGE YOU WISH TO SEE IN THE WORLD."
–*Mahatma Gandhi, Activist, Humanitarian and Global Peacemaker*

Global peace starts by fostering peace inside you. When there is peace in every individual, there can't help but be peace on the planet. Like all change, it must start from within.

As you begin to incorporate the principles in this book, you will notice a shift in your own inner landscape. You will begin to cultivate more inner peace. With those personal choices, comes a more peaceful life, more peaceful experiences, more peaceful friends and associates and soon, a more peaceful planet.

Conclusion

"You may say I'm a dreamer... but I'm not the only one. I hope someday you'll join us... and the world will live as one."
–*John Lennon, Singer, Songwriter, Musician and Social Activist*

Imagine a world where people from all walks of life and all corners of the globe have access to healthy food, clothing, shelter, running water, electricity, Internet, an authentic education and all the basics of life.

In this place, humanity has risen to a level of awakened consciousness where never again does one human being cause hurt or harm to another human being or to our precious home, Mother Earth.

The news stories that fill the airwaves speak of the incredible expansion and elevation happening on the planet. Global warming and the destruction of each other, our oceans, forests and animal brothers and sisters are a thing of the past.

In this new global society, healthy organic living food restaurants replace junk food restaurants on every street corner. You don't need to ask where the organic section of the produce department is when you visit a store because all the "chemically ladened, toxic GMO" produce isn't an option anymore. Solar panels and other renewable resources fuel our vehicles, homes and technical devices so there is no need to rob Mother Earth of her blood (oil) and no need to start wars that fight over who owns it. Peace, generosity and love become the natural state of being on our planet.

A new educational system emerges based on creativity, imagination and interest instead of rote memorization. These schools fuel the genius minds and hearts of all students who enter their halls. Graduates go on to create careers that excite and enliven them and contribute to the wellbeing of society in remarkable ways.

People now make their living doing what they love and share their unique gifts and talents for a world that appreciates them and compensates them accordingly and amply.

In this scenario, health care becomes true to its name. Because people are now properly nourished, exercised and naturally healthy, there is no need for a purple pill that counter balances the yellow pill that compensates for the side effects of the red pill.

Insurance will do what it was meant to do, help keep people healthy, naturally. Instead of paying for pharmaceuticals that contribute to the decline in health, they now provide coverage for cutting edge healing technologies (such as those we discussed in chapter 2, HEAL), that detox, heal and youth the body without harmful side effects. These newly revised insurance policies now cover healing, detoxing, anti-aging, natural treatments that help people not only feel younger and healthier but look younger and healthier as well.

Think about it, healthier people means a healthier economy, a healthier country and a healthier planet. It also means more productivity and greater expressions of imagination allowing for the creation of new and exciting discoveries that help make our lives and our world better.

Playing In the Vortex

The fountain of youth is not a place; it is a state of being and level of consciousness. I call this state of being, the vortex. Many people refer to it as "being in the zone." Everything is possible here. And when you place yourself in this state of being, you are forever radiant and youthful.

Athletes, actors, speakers and others who have experienced being in the zone, speak of that magical moment when something greater then them is working through them. In this state, you are invincible, undeniable and super human.

I have experienced being in the vortex countless times, speaking and dancing on stage and have witnessed others being elevated into its opulent potentiality as well.

Dancing in the Zone

Every once in a while you meet someone who is so rich in light and love that you just want to be around them. My dear friend and colleague, Tor Campbell, is one of those people. Tor is a magnificent dancer, singer, teacher and choreographer. But his real gift is sharing his brilliant light with others.

Every time Tor teaches, his classes are packed to the brim with enthusiastic students. He is doing much more than giving these students a workout. He is literally scooping them up in his energy field and transporting them into the vortex of infinite possibilities. His students rave, "I have never danced so well in my life," and "I've never been able to move like that before. But, somehow, in Tor's class, I can." It's no wonder he has them lining up out the door to take his class. Tor's light and love are so powerful that he literally creates a vortex of energy that transports each student into the higher realms where everything is possible. This vortex is where the real magic and miracles of our life occur.

Now, you can enter into this field of infinite possibilities anytime you wish. Just grab hold of one or more of these keys I have given you. They hold the power to magically transport you through the portal gateway and into the fountain of youth where everything is possible.

When you apply the keys in this book, Spirit can step in and use you to create such beauty, genius, healing and love that it's beyond what you could comprehend as humanly possible. And, the by-products of allowing Spirit to flow through you in contribution to others are eternal youthfulness, radiance, beauty and sex appeal.

People call these experiences miracles. But the truth is they're simply everyday occurrences that are available to us at every moment when we choose to embrace this way of life.

Everyone doesn't have to:

- Workout 2-3 hours a day
- Eat 100% organic living foods
- Continuously partake of 100% natural detox treatments
- Perform daily spiritual practices
- Open their heart up to the entire world...

Not everyone wants to.

However, if everyone just took one step in the direction of these key practices, they would certainly live healthier, happier and more fulfilled lives.

If one person wakes up after reading this book and feels better about circling the sun each year, if one person is inspired to live their purpose and passion and shine their light in the world, then the book has done its job.

I invite you to take what works and know that there is a better way. Instead of believing that aging is your only option, know that you can choose youthfulness and all the incredible blessings that accompany this choice.

I encourage you to go on an adventure to discover the beauty of your own being; body, mind, heart, soul and spirit, and allow that to serve you in your purpose on this planet.

Wishing you a life filled with miracles. Know that you can be absolutely undeniably radiant, beautiful, youthful and sexy at every stage in your life. I look forward to eternally skinny dipping in the fountain of youth with you!

Acknowledgments

One of the greatest blessings of skinny dipping in the fountain of youth is the overflowing love and incredible connections with others that this path affords you. I could fill an entire book with the names of angels who have touched my life for the better.

If we've ever crossed paths and shared a smile and a kind word somewhere upon life's journey, be it on an airplane, the dance floor, a conference, etc., I thank you for blessing me with a little piece of your heart and soul. Know that our encounter has left me greater for having met you.

A very special thank you to my amazing book editor Carol Skeldon and my incredible graphic artist, photographer and book designer, Harrison G. McKoy. You are both my treasured friends and your hours of dedication, generosity, extraordinary talents and creative contributions have blessed this book beyond measure. You are the reason it is in physical form today.

An enormous heartfelt thank you to my remarkable teacher, Vicki Reiner. Your patience, generosity and wisdom have blessed me tremendously. Thank you for the gift of "sight."

My profound gratitude and appreciation to my amazing angel, Jill Marcel Wittenmyer. Your incredible love, guidance and generous support has literally been the wind beneath my wings.

To my precious friends, Laurie Wilder and Ray Davis, a very special thank you for continuously and generously opening your hearts and home to me. Your love is a powerful source of joy and inspiration in my life.

To all my extraordinary teachers and mentors who are also my treasured friends, thank you for sharing your wisdom with me; Rev. Vicki Reiner, Jill Marcel Wittenmyer, Mrs. Rose Nack, Mrs. Jacobs, Dr. Michael Beckwith, Dr. Joanne Coleman, Dr. Sonia Powers, Rev. Cheryl Ward, Rev. Coco Stewart, Katherine Woodward Thomas, Claire Zammit, Dr. Michele Meiche, Nina Kellogg, Norman Cohen, Cameron Thor, Kaya Redford and Dr. Julie Ann Cohn.

I am incredibly grateful to all of my extraordinary confidants and cheerleaders, who have been with me through every step of the way; Gail Larkin, Carolina (Cookie) Carosella, Carol Skeldon, Lynn Banfi, Jill Marcel Wittenmyer, Laurie Wilder, Ray Davis, Naimah Al-waajid and my mother, Lucille. Your precious love and unending support have kept me going through this exciting and arduous journey. You each mean the world to me.

To my sweet friend, Kelly Sullivan Walden, thank you for generously giving birth to the title of my book through the power of your intentional dreams.

A huge thank you to my incredibly loving and talented clairvoyant confidants, Kelly McCormick, Diana Bernas and Tasha Rae. Your words continue to be a source of tremendous healing and expansion. I treasure each one of you.

My deep appreciation to my amazing literary agent, Devra Jacobs. Your loving support and generosity of the heart are astounding.

A tremendous thank you to my hairstylist, trainer and dear friend, Aitch G. McKoy who always makes me look and feel my best and my trainers and close friends, Ricky Johnson and Dani Scherrer. Thank you all for assisting me in the gym, proving gravity wrong and helping me teach others that working out is an imperative part of growing young.

Thank you to my sweet friends who have blessed me along the way, each one of you is a precious gift to me; Maribel Smith, Danny Davalos, Dr. Elena Pezzini, Tyreese Washington, TJ Storm, Cynthia Kersey, Rick Mars, Tammy Miller-Mars, Johanna Hulme, Steve Sedlic, Jarvis Essex, Diana Presley, Lori Hart, Zoe Vincent, David Boufford, Sheronda Lewis, David Powell, Idris Hester, Julian Michael, Mimi Kirk, Victor Hugo Saavedra, Happy Oasis, Dee Upshaw, Desire Bartlett, Rosie Tos, Nichole LeShawn Woods, Rerani Taurima, Denise Lampron, Joelene Walker, Alex Stephens, Debra Hockemeyer and Susan Reiner.

Immense thanks to my photographers assistants, Laurie Wilder and Tyreese Washington. Your support during our photoshoot was immeasurable.

To each one of my precious friends from my four incredible communities, Agape, Salsa Familia, Raw Food, Gold's Gym and my Clairvoyant Class, I love and appreciate each one of you and your beautiful presence in my life.

Last but not least, to my beloved family, a very special thank you:

To my Mother, Lucille; your outer beauty is exceeded only by your inner beauty. At nearly eighty years young, you continue to show me what it really looks like to eternally skinny dip in the fountain of youth.

To my father, who gave me my love for words, knowledge and language.

To my sisters, Katerina, who keeps me "polished," Suzanne, who always dots my 'i's" and crosses my "t's" and Christine, who keeps me stylish and current. Your love, kindness and unending support mean the world to me.

To my new brothers (my sisters' husbands) Dan and Walt, who teach me by example what it looks like to be an extraordinary man.

To my beloved brother, Mark who is now my true angel. Thank you for showing me what real courage and love looks like.

And, to God, the Infinite Universal Source of Light and Love, for this precious and breathtaking gift called Life.

Book Credits

Cover Designer, Book Layout, Photographer
Harrison G. McKoy

Back Cover Photographer
Cyrus Marshall

Assistant Photographers
Tyreese Washington
Laurie Wilder

Location
Ray Davis
Laurie Wilder

Stylists
Gail Larkin
Christine Inda

Hair Stylist
Aitch G. McKoy

Editor
Carol Skeldon

Executive Producers
Dr. Gregory and Lucille Rochetta Inda

.

The Author

Dr. Elizabeth is an inspirational speaker, talk show host, brand ambassador and author.

She holds two undergraduate degrees from Loyola Marymount University and a Doctorate in Dentistry from University of the Pacific in San Francisco. She is Board Certified in the State of California.

Dr. Elizabeth has been a keynote speaker at many prestigious international conferences as well as a guest expert on numerous television and radio shows. She teaches men and women alike how to be undeniably radiant, beautiful, youthful and sexy at every age.

Dr. Elizabeth is the host and creator of the "The Dr Elizabeth Show" airing on YouTube and iTunes Podcast.

In addition to her extensive medical and spiritual background, Dr. Elizabeth has studied whole living foods, meditation, elite fitness training and intuitive intelligence. These art forms endow the work she does with individuals and groups, speaking at conferences and events and leading international retreats to exotic locations around the world.

Dr. Elizabeth welcomes you to join her on this exciting adventure of skinny dipping in the fountain of youth. Dive in… the water's Divine!

For more info please visit www.DrElizabeth.com

CPSIA information can be obtained
at www.ICGtesting.com
Printed in the USA
LVHW022024030620
657308LV00021B/2234